THE
POWER
IN THE
MIDDLE

THE
POWER
IN THE
MIDDLE

Navigating Your Midlife with Confidence

ELIZABETH O'BRIEN

BLOOMSBURY ACADEMIC
NEW YORK • LONDON • OXFORD • NEW DELHI • SYDNEY

BLOOMSBURY ACADEMIC
Bloomsbury Publishing Inc, 1385 Broadway, New York, NY 10018, USA
Bloomsbury Publishing Plc, 50 Bedford Square, London, WC1B 3DP, UK
Bloomsbury Publishing Ireland, 29 Earlsfort Terrace, Dublin 2, D02 AY28, Ireland

BLOOMSBURY, BLOOMSBURY ACADEMIC and the Diana logo
are trademarks of Bloomsbury Publishing Plc

First published in the United States of America 2025

Copyright © Bloomsbury Publishing, Inc., 2025

All images courtesy of Reagan Harrold

Moon River
from the Paramount Pictures feature film BREAKFAST AT TIFFANY'S
Words by Johnny Mercer
Music by Henry Mancini
Copyright © 1961 Sony Music Publishing (US) LLC
Copyright Renewed
All Rights Administered by Sony Music Publishing (US) LLC,
424 Church Street, Suite 1200, Nashville, TN 37219
International Copyright Secured All Rights Reserved
Reprinted by Permission of Hal Leonard LLC

All rights reserved. No part of this publication may be: i) reproduced or transmitted in any form, electronic or mechanical, including photocopying, recording or by means of any information storage or retrieval system without prior permission in writing from the publishers; or ii) used or reproduced in any way for the training, development or operation of artificial intelligence (AI) technologies, including generative AI technologies. The rights holders expressly reserve this publication from the text and data mining exception as per Article 4(3) of the Digital Single Market Directive (EU) 2019/790.

Bloomsbury Publishing Inc does not have any control over, or responsibility for, any third-party websites referred to or in this book. All internet addresses given in this book were correct at the time of going to press. The author and publisher regret any inconvenience caused if addresses have changed or sites have ceased to exist, but can accept no responsibility for any such changes.

Library of Congress Cataloging-in-Publication Data Available

ISBN: HB: 979-8-8818-0579-1
eBook: 979-8-8818-0580-7

Typeset by Susan Ramundo
Printed and bound in the USA, by Integrated Books International

For product safety related questions contact productsafety@bloomsbury.com.

To find out more about our authors and books visit www.bloomsbury.com
and sign up for our newsletters.

CONTENTS

Preface — vii
Acknowledgments — xix

1. Feeling Stuck in Midlife — 1
2. Redefining Wellness — 21
3. Mental and Emotional Health — 39
4. Physical Health — 55
5. Appearance — 77
6. Intimate Relationships — 95
7. Social Health — 117
8. Vocation — 141
9. Leisure — 163
10. Belief Systems and Spiritual Health — 181

Conclusion — 199
References — 203
Index — 209
About the Author — 225

PREFACE

I was sitting in my academic office with my graduate school mentor discussing his impending move to my college town. We were chatting about life and work challenges, what we'd both been doing personally and professionally during the last few years. I shared with him some of the reasons that I'd made certain life decisions based on my family life and professional expectations. He looked at me and said, "Isn't it interesting how you've become cautious as you've gotten older? Some of that happens by the necessity of getting older and wiser, and some of it happens because we become comfortable in our surroundings. I'm surprised by this because, in my memory of you, you used to be fearless."

I remember the sinking feeling that followed when he said that, knowing that he was right. I had been fearless in my younger adulthood, often taking risks without worrying about the consequences because it didn't occur to me that I would fail. My father often used the word *insouciant* to describe my manner, a word that means showing a casual lack of concern. It wasn't that I didn't care about what I was doing; rather it was because I was willing to take risks with little concern about the possible adverse consequences to myself. Call it a lack of experience and resources, but with youth on my side, personal and professional risks in my mid-twenties seemed to surround me; I was new at everything, so why not try any- and everything?

But experiences and aging have a way of teaching us important lessons and helping us to home in on staying safe. The damage caused by failures and false starts have a way of teaching us what we're good at and what we're not, and as humans, we tend to gravitate toward positive reinforcements, the things that reinforce our positive attributes and reward us for certain behaviors. Are you good at school? You can get lots of degrees and get a job. Are you good at networking? You can become a successful businesswoman and entrepreneur. Are you good at nurturing others? You can become a successful parent and bring forth the next generation.

When we start our lives, the possibilities seem endless, but as we progress on our journey, we may likely find that we've narrowed our range of experiences. This narrowing can create limits in our lives that may help to keep us content and safe, but limits may result in less stimulation and risk. In my case, my mentor commented that I had stayed in my current professional position for longer than anticipated, and he attributed that to my fearfulness about changing my life, even though I had the potential to take risks and take on other professional challenges.

He wasn't wrong; I had become careful. There were things that I was afraid to lose at this stage of my life: the stability of my income, the autonomy of controlling my work life, contentment in my marriage, my ability to support my aging parents, the list goes on. I had filled my life and résumé with tasks and roles that looked like success from the outside, but on the inside, I knew those achievements masked a real fear of truly breaking free of inertia and doing something that felt *different*. I knew that I felt stuck and that I'd been living with that feeling for a while, but I was not sure what it would take to create change. It was as if I were protecting myself with layers of tasks, professional successes, and safety, which was obscuring my true self, the person I am at my core.

WHAT DOES EVERY WOMAN WANT?

Over drinks with girlfriends one evening, I spoke about my mentor's comments and how I felt. They did what good friends do: they listened, they grew defensive on my behalf, and then they asked hard questions. The unanswered questions and feelings I was experiencing were circling their minds too. The commonality they shared with me was a general feeling of awkwardness; they had worked hard to get to specific places in their lives, with family, friends, jobs, and in their own skin, but they still felt that something was off or missing. Instead of feeling a sense of freedom, peace, and joy, they were wrestling with an existential angst that they couldn't quite put their fingers on. It felt good to not be alone, but it also left me wondering how we had ended up in this place. I make it a habit to surround myself with smart women I admire, and if they were struggling, what hope was there for me?

The intangible thing that we all seemed to want was to feel confident and content with who we are. We want to be comfortable in our skin and to know that we are competent to handle the surprises that life throws at us. We want to reconsider the "why" behind the way in which we'd been living our lives and confirm if that was still our why—if it was something we still value. And if the ideas we had valued before were no longer working for us, what do we value now? We want to acknowledge the hard work we'd put in to gain our experiences and recognize that our failures and successes taught us enough about our resilience to keep moving forward in our lives, taking risks that make us uncomfortable, and stretching ourselves in ways our younger selves wouldn't have even considered.

What was it about this stage of our lives that made these questions seem so important? And why is it that many of us found ourselves questioning our values or how we expressed our values at this point? The answer seemed to be where we found ourselves in our life stage: midlife.

MIDLIFE AND DEVELOPMENT

In my work as a college professor, one of the classes that I have developed and taught for counselors is human development. I've always thought that I would write a book on human development that delves into lifespan with a slightly different spin, but the challenge with that topic is that it's been done a lot. In college, most of the classes on development center on the early years, from fetus to early adulthood (age twenty-five or so), because that's where the "action" is. There are so many interesting and rapid changes that we experience during the first twenty-five years of our lives, but once we hit the adulthood mark, changes appear to slow down considerably. During the middle and later adult years, we evolve more slowly, and we often receive our cues for how our lives will progress based on family expectations, social norms from peers and popular culture, or through our community (Broderick & Blewitt, 2006, p. 404).

I've often thought it would be nice if my life came with a guidebook that provided some general parameters about what to expect at certain stages and phases and how to navigate those changes as the most functional version of myself. When I imagined creating a book about human development, I thought it would be a traditional textbook with more therapeutic interventions woven through it. What I realized is that I am far more passionate about writing a version of a guidebook specifically for women as we enter our middle years: what you can expect at this stage of your development and how to navigate the issues you encounter successfully. I imagine it very similarly to how I work with clients in my therapeutic space: some education about what is happening, some solid questions to get you thinking and reflecting more deeply about what is going on and how you think about the issues, and some thoughts about how you might move forward in your journey through these common issues. As I write these pages, I'm imagining you as though you are sitting in my therapy room. We're having a conversation about the struggles that you find yourself encountering as you traverse this stage of your life, and we work together to find out how you want to move through this new, uncharted territory of your development.

So I took a risk and started writing this book, which will help you—and me—tackle our development through midlife as women. Most of what you're experiencing is totally normal for you. You are a unique individual and what is normal for you is not going to be normal for your sister, your friend, your coworker, or your pharmacist. I'm going to give you some general guidelines to work with. Some of them are going to be on target and some of them are not going to be as precise for you. That's okay; the point is to get you thinking about what you might be able to expect. Some of what is in these pages will work for you and some might not. This is very similar to any other stage of development—not everyone goes through the same process in the same way. That said, having a frame of reference for what may be "typical" can help us all to have a notion of what to expect and a greater perceived level of control when we encounter developmental changes that are new or different from what we've experienced previously. But the question remains, what makes midlife so different?

Midlife is a stage that is full of biological, social, and emotional evolution; however, these changes aren't discussed openly. I had a very wise professor in college (not the mentor mentioned earlier) who used to say that there are some things that we're prepared for in our heads but not in our hearts. I think that there is a great deal of truth to her statement as it relates to our midlife development. We know as women there will be changes: in our heads we are intellectually prepared for inevitable transformations, the physical changes to our bodies, the emotional changes that we navigate as we deal with more complex issues with our families and loved ones as they change, the social changes that occur as we become the more experienced people in the room rather than the newbies, and so forth. Some of these changes are exciting and fun; it's nice to be able to mentor people who want to learn from you. Some of them are less fun, like looking down at your phone camera and seeing your neck sagging. (I will never forget the first time I saw that—pure shock!) In my head, I knew that with age comes both wisdom and sagging, but my heart was not prepared for the realities as they had begun to reveal themselves.

Midlife development for women is compounded by the hormonal changes that occur as we move into perimenopause and menopause. Although men can experience hormonal shifts in midlife, women's experiences can be more pronounced and are also tied to our reproduction, which for many is at the heart of femininity and the value we place on ourselves and how culture values us (Broderick & Blewitt, 2006, p. 412). Although many women don't necessarily identify menopause as the number one issue that they have to traverse in midlife, it can have a profound effect on overall functioning (hormones are very powerful) in terms of emotions and cognition (Thomas, Mitchell, & Woods, 2018).

Additional events that also absorb our attention in midlife include attending to marriages/partnerships, raising children into their middle childhood and adolescent years, helping aging parents or relatives navigate healthcare or other age-related issues, managing resources in light of multiple and increasing demands, grappling with existential and spiritual questions as we deal with our mortality, managing our changing bodies, general health, and abilities as our bodies age, and navigating our jobs or careers as we mature into our roles or consider new or different ventures.

When we're younger, we expect that we will go through periods marked by a great deal of development and upheaval—finding partners, having children, making big moves. But as we become settled into our lives and the rhythm of consistency, we can forget that the dynamics of change are something that our minds and bodies crave and that if we don't seek out unique experiences, then we may begin to feel flat or uninspired. I have worked with many women who say to me, "I'm too old to start something new; if I were at a different place in my life, I would think differently." These are the same women who come to counseling feeling stuck and mired in their inability to "shake things up" in their lives in a way that changes their perspective. The issue with thinking we're "too old" is that we're as young as we're ever going to be and there is no such thing as perfect timing. If we don't take our opportunities when we have them, we may lose them.

What we forget is that we're humans in evolution every day until the day we stop breathing. When we as women do the same things over and over because they worked for us in the past or because they cloak us in a feeling of safety, we begin to feel discomfort or angst. This can occur because we are living within the values, beliefs, and behaviors that worked for us in the past but may no longer be serving us. Whereas our values, beliefs, and behaviors fit us in the past—much like a beloved pair of jeans—it doesn't mean that they fit or work the same way they did when we were younger. As an example, Casey was a midlife woman who worked in nonprofit management for more than two decades. She enjoyed building these businesses from the ground up, and when they were successful, she moved on to the next big project. As she approached her early fifties, she realized how tired and stretched she felt. She was trying to continuously build successful nonprofits while also tending to her personal life. At the age and stage that she found herself, working sixteen-hour days and building new businesses while also being present for her children and partner was asking a lot. In our work together, Casey began to realize that her resistance to staying at the same nonprofit past the point of initial success was rooted in her belief that if she wasn't solving problems or building a company, she was stagnant. Anyone who has worked in the day-to-day world of nonprofit management knows that the problem-solving that needs to happen daily to keep things moving is far from boring or stagnant. But Casey's belief that unless she was in triage mode, she was stagnant was also keeping her from a life of work stability, which would make it possible to show up for her personal life. She was exhausted and had a hard time admitting that not only did she not have the same level of interest in working to build a new nonprofit, but she also didn't have the same stamina that she did in her early thirties.

Using a series of exercises and questions, we worked through how her work-life values in her earlier career had served her well and helped her build success and competence. We also discussed how those same values were sabotaging other areas of her life at this stage, specifically her relationship with her children and partner. After considering what she wanted for herself in her personal life and how she wanted to take care of her physical and mental health, Casey committed to remaining at her current nonprofit job for eighteen months to "try out" what it was like to be a veteran employee rather than a nonprofit builder so that she could lean into her value of prioritizing family and health at this stage of her life. Although this switch seems as though it would be easy for many, it took a great deal of self-reflection and time for Casey to refocus herself on her reprioritized value of family first rather than building her career. This example is just one of the many that women in midlife juggle, figuring out what we value, how we prioritize what we say we value, and then engaging in the behaviors that reflect us living those values.

IS THERE A SOLUTION?

Like Casey, you are likely in a place in your life where you realize that some of the values, beliefs, and behaviors that brought you to this place in your life may not be the same values that will move you forward into the next phase of your life. Midlife is an opportunity to take stock and become a more refined version of yourself. What do I mean by this? *Refining* is a term used to discuss the process of extracting a mineral or compound from a natural resource. Think about sugar. To get the sugar that we use for cooking and baking, we first grow cane, separate the sugar compound from the plant, convert it to usable substance, and finally purify it to create the sugar that is used in cooking. Your development and growth are very much like that process. Every experience that you have can give you more information about who you are and what you value. The more time you spend reflecting on the impact of important experiences (extracting the meaning) and converting your insights into practice (by modifying or changing your thinking, behaving, and emotions based on the insight), the more refined and truer version of yourself you become. When you move into the midpoint of your life, you've had many opportunities that teach you about yourself; you've chosen to change or not change based on these insights; and you've refined yourself for your early adult years. At this point in your life, the work is twofold: engaging in a self-inventory and also removing outer, protective layers that may obscure your true essence at this stage of your life. Taking the time to reflect and inventory your life to this point and then to anticipate how you may need to adapt based on the next phase of your life is part of the refining process. It is you in your truest and purest form, the version of you that is wholly aligned with your values and beliefs.

What I have found when women embark on this path of self-reflection and refinement is a sense of ease with who and how they are in the world. This ease comes from self-knowledge and understanding that accepting oneself is the highest form of self-love. You've met these women. They are sure of themselves and can shrug off other people's perceptions of them, they have strong boundaries, and they stay true to what they value. They know that living in this alignment doesn't mean that anyone else is less than, nor are they less than for living their values. Rather, they know what works for them and honor that by staying true to those values and respecting other women for living their truth, knowing that someone else living their truth doesn't threaten the way they live their life. This is true power—a type of power that we can truly harness in midlife.

I don't know about you, but the woman described above is the person who I strive to be, and I think it takes a lot of work and personal inventory to become my version of her. That's the point of this book: what is the midlife, refined version of you that you want to become? I find that when I am working toward refining myself, I should concentrate on the things that I can do, rather than punishing myself for the things that I need to stop. What do I mean by that? I think that one of the ways that we work to become our refined selves is to reassess areas in our lives that we can control and to define for ourselves what health in those areas should look like for us. Let's start with what we can control, where we may feel stuck, and shake up our previously held beliefs about who we are and work to refine ourselves.

THE PUREST VERSION OF YOURSELF

As you read this book, you'll notice the focus on wellness. Wellness is more than the absence of illness; it is the active movement toward being healthy. When we focus on our personal wellness, not only are we engaging in activities that we can control, but we are also creating space for the most refined and best version of ourselves. I hear the sighs right now. "Ugh, it's another book about wellness!" Yes and no. It is a book about wellness and it's also a book about what wellness can look like in midlife. This work is about confronting beliefs that we inherit from others (read: family, society, social media, etc.), removing the layers of expectations or protections with which we have cloaked ourselves, and determining if these are best for us as the refined version of ourselves in midlife. It's also about confronting reality. Spoiler alert: we're all going to die and since our time is finite (more so now than twenty years ago), we need to take responsibility for what we can control and be proactive in living our truest life now, not waiting until it's convenient. Second spoiler alert: life is rarely convenient.

So here's how this book will help. We're going to look at eight different areas in our lives and seek our truest, most refined version of personal wellness in each area. In this way, we will seek and find a more refined version of ourselves, filled with the wisdom of our experiences and living within the values that are true to who we are and who we want to be at this stage of our lives. Wellness literature in counseling is based on the research of Myers and Sweeney (2004), who devised a model of wellness called the "Indivisible Self," which conceptualizes wellness in terms of five life tasks—work, leisure, friendship, love, and spirit—along with five additional factors, which make up the "Indivisible Self," including the essential self, social self, creative self, physical self, and coping self. This model serves as a starting point for the chapters in this book, many of which align with the Indivisible Self model of wellness.

These chapters provide information about current trends on each topic and how these infiltrate popular culture. Additionally, each chapter contains exercises and reflection questions that are intended to help you determine your baseline of wellness in each area and what you may want to consider doing differently or keeping the same. When people think about wellness, they often think about mental health and physical wellness, and I certainly discuss those. I also look at both intimate relationships and social health, which many believe are the same but have some distinct characteristics. I look at how spiritual health and belief systems are important at this stage of life, especially when considering existential questions about the meaning of life and how we navigate our wounds. I also take a deeper look at vocation (career) and leisure (who has time for that?) to see the role that these play in our ongoing development. Finally, I also take some time to examine our appearance and how changes in our bodies, how we perceive ourselves, and how the world perceives us can impact how we move through our middle years and beyond. In each chapter, you are asked to reflect on your values, assumptions/beliefs, and behaviors; to self-assess whether those are still working for you; and to decide how you want to live now and in the future. Again, our process is about refining who we are to distill the clearest and purest versions of ourselves. The purpose of these reflections is to quiet the noise of others, to help you clarify your thoughts, and to get in touch with your true self.

DISCLAIMER

As I write this book, I imagine you, my reader, as if you are sitting in my counseling room, but there are limits to this allusion. Yes, I am a trained counselor with more than twenty years of experience working with individuals across the lifespan in many different settings. I write this book with the aspiration of giving you a mix of scientific facts and information from scholarly literature, posing questions to get you thinking, and pulling from my experiences as a therapist. I also completed interviews with midlife women as part of this work; note that I use pseudonyms to protect the privacy of individuals when requested.

As a counselor, I am trained to help people navigate challenges that naturally occur as they change and develop. Counseling is based on a wellness perspective with a belief that although individuals have the inherent strengths and resources to work through many issues, sometimes external help is needed to gain a different perspective on one's problems. This book is written in that paradigm, that by examining wellness and what you can control you will rediscover or find the tools that you need to successfully navigate the challenges of midlife.

That said, a book is not a person. If you find that the challenges that you face are bigger than one (or more) self-help book can manage, then there is wisdom in talking to someone else about what is going on in your life. This could be a friend, family member, or trusted confidant. Please remember that there is something very freeing in speaking with someone who is a trained helping professional who is not directly involved in your life to give you some much-needed perspective and guidance. Readings, podcasts, and other digestible pieces of information can be great resources for growth, and sometimes they are a precursor to a deeper dive into your psyche, such as going to counseling or seeking more intensive treatment.

There may be aspects of this book that you find triggering; thinking and reflecting on your wellness—your autonomy to control your life, people, or past events that influence how you feel about yourself—can sometimes have unpredictable influence on your mental well-being. If you find that occurs, then please seek mental health or medical treatment as needed. The 988 Suicide & Crisis Lifeline is a resource that can be invaluable to you if you find yourself in crisis. I know some of my readers are thinking that this is rather deep for a book about changes in midlife; however, I also know that since I am not there with you as you read this, it is better that I prepare you for as many eventualities as possible. That said, I hope this experience is more reflective and thoughtful work than painful.

A final thought as you begin this book: I am many things, and I have lots of opinions about many things. I am going to write from my lens as a trained professional counselor on subjects for which I am not a subject matter expert. I know mental health and I know how struggles in developmental life stages can manifest in the therapy room, and I discuss things like physical health, spiritual health, and leisure from that lens. That doesn't mean that I have specialized training as a fitness coach, a minister, or an activity therapist. It does mean that I've completed research to give you the best information that I can with my training as a mental health counselor about how these aspects of wellness can impact your development.

I'm excited and I hope you are too! Let's start doing the internal work of refining who we are to become the best versions of ourselves as we move into this new (to us) phase of our lives. There is power midlife, and it is ours for the taking.

ACKNOWLEDGMENTS

It certainly takes a village of people to make dreams and projects a reality, and this book is no different. First, I want to thank my readers for picking this book out of the many that you have to choose from. Your interest and support mean the world to me!

Many years ago, when I interviewed at University of Tennessee–Chattanooga, I was told that I could create the career that I wanted. I took them at their word and have had the opportunity to grow as a teacher, scholar, counselor, and leader. I am exceptionally grateful for the colleagues, friends, and students that I have met through this community. Thank you to Ariel Curry, my book coach and consultant, for helping me to make this book a reality. Your balance of enthusiasm and tough love through this process is most appreciated. And to Peyton Gwaltney, my marketing and social media guide, I appreciate your patience and every pep talk you were willing to give me. I'll likely need more pep talks, so keep them coming.

Thank you to my editorial team at Rowman & Littlefield/Bloomsbury Publishing. Jonathan Joyce, thanks for the book light, the book deal, and the reassurance that there really was a book deal. May we work on more projects in the future. Sarah Rinehart, thank you for your patience, which you seem to have in spades. To Erin McGarvey, if I could meet you in person, I would buy you coffee and a pastry and proceed to thank you profusely for making this book infinitely more readable. And to folks on the team whom I haven't met but who have brought this book to completion, thank you.

To all my dear friends and family who asked, "How's the writing going?" Those check-ins were an important part of holding me accountable, encouraging me, and showing how much you care. I am so glad to have cultivated such a strong support system and I hope that I show you the same encouragement that you give me.

To my dear friend and first reader, Amy Gruber, the first person I told about this book idea, for your tireless cheerleading, your willingness to answer every question, and for reading every *ugly* first draft. This book really wouldn't have happened without you.

To my sweet Woodrow, the heartbeat at my feet. I've been told it isn't scholarly or professional to thank a dog for support, but it's my book and I'll do what I want. Extra treats for you to make up for all the lost walks and playtime that writing took.

To my parents, Hans and Carolyn O'Brien. I am acutely aware of how fortunate I am to have supportive parents who gave me the latitude and freedom (within reason) to grow into the adult that I've become. The life I have wouldn't have happened without you.

To my husband, Kyle, for your support, counsel, patience, and love. I couldn't pick a better companion to travel through this life—on to the next adventure!

CHAPTER ONE

FEELING STUCK IN MIDLIFE

When I decided to have a midlife crisis and attempted to burn down my life, I told my husband I wasn't sure I wanted to be married any longer, I stopped taking my parents' phone calls, I started looking for a different job, and I researched tiny houses—the whole privileged twenty-first-century stereotype. The entire crisis culminated with me in an ashram in the North Carolina wilderness for seventy-two hours of complete silence, vegan food, and meditation (seriously, the *entire* stereotype). It was my very own low-budget version of *Eat, Pray, Love*. Reading this situated in one paragraph, it sounds like a short-term, tumultuous couple of months; the reality is that the slow burn of personal discontent began long before I ended up in a meditation circle filled with other women in the isolated wilderness.

Lots of women go through some version of this story, though theirs may be more or less extreme than my example. As we get caught in the hustle of living our everyday lives, tending to our families, friends, jobs, homes, health, hobbies, spiritual lives, and additional commitments, we can find ourselves exhausted and overwhelmed, wondering if the hamster wheels that we can't seem to jump off are our actual lives. In my counseling room, I've heard countless women say, "Is this it?!?" and then apologize immediately for asking the question because they believe that they appear ungrateful. How dare we not enjoy tending to a multitude of life responsibilities that outweigh our personal rights to feeling fulfilled as individuals! I certainly understand that feeling. I love all the opportunities that I have in my life caring for the people I love and playing my role in the world. But, at the end of the day, when I sat alone with my thoughts, I too had to ask myself the question, *is this it?* And—if I feel as though it is sucking the life and personhood out of me—*is it still worth it?*

For most women, it's not worth it. It wasn't worth it to me (see paragraph 1), and for lack of any other thoughtful solution, we often try anything to create change to help us get unstuck and feel more at ease. The need for relief from mental and emotional discomfort can lead people to engage in impulsive decisions that lack forethought and create even more disruption and chaos than what they are already experiencing (again, I refer you to paragraph 1).

In counseling sessions with my clients, I often tell them that blame is not a useful concept. Blame doesn't help solve the problem; it allows individuals to scapegoat other people or responsibilities for the real issue, robbing individuals of the ability to become active problem solvers in their own lives. So, if paragraph 1 or some variation of it seems familiar to you, don't blame your past self for the impulsive decisions you've made to solve the problem of midlife unhappiness. The reality is that you were likely attempting to solve a new problem in an old way, and although those old ways of solving problems were useful in the past, the solution to reimagining your life and happiness at this stage won't be achieved with a new haircut. It is going to take time and reflection to consider who you are now and how you want to live in a way that fits with the person you are now.

One problem that you may grapple with is that you are living in the values, beliefs, and boundaries that worked for you in the past but likely are not working for you now. Our old values, beliefs, and boundaries served a function for our past selves; they were good for the time and space when they were created. As we evolve, we may find that either what we value shifts or the way we express our values has shifted. This may be for a variety of reasons, including that we have collected more experiences that inform our beliefs about the world or that our boundaries around our values and beliefs have shifted. We explore these ideas more in the next section.

THE PROBLEM

Likely you picked up this book because you are uncomfortable or have identified your life stage as a culprit for why you are experiencing emotions that can range from a sense of ennui to exhaustion to anger. As you reflect on how you are living your life now, you may realize that you have "outgrown" your old values, beliefs, and boundaries, which no longer work for you as they did in the past. Perhaps these values, beliefs, and boundaries need reevaluation and retooling. The good news is that most women go through a self-evaluation during the midlife stage, which can range from small tweaks to a complete "teardown." Yours may not be of the "burn it down" variety, but rather in particular parts of your life, like your family life or marriage, your work, or your friendships. Whether a modification of specific areas of your life or a holistic evaluation, it is important to note that there may be generational differences in how you're experiencing this midlife shift and reevaluation. Let's explore the women who came before us and how our experiences may be influenced by theirs.

Okay, Boomer

Although their generation is the butt of many jokes, the women of the baby boomer generation did blaze a trail, by virtue of its sheer size and the good luck of being born during an affluent economic cycle. Companies and services tailored goods and opportunities to these women in ways that were unprecedented in previous generations. This is also the generation of women who moved into middle age in the 1980s and 1990s after Betty Friedan's *Feminine Mystique* guided the second wave of feminism in the 1960s and 1970s. The results of this second wave of feminism resulted in legislation that guided women's choices through the 1980s on such issues as civil rights and women's rights for employment, reproductive rights (such as access to contraceptives and abortions), and financial independence without male relatives as cosigners. These innovations had the potential to liberate women's abilities to live to their full potential with a (seemingly) endless array of possibilities for the future. The corollary to these accomplishments is that rights were secured predominantly for white, educated, middle-class women. Women's roadblocks are often termed the "glass ceiling," and in this case, the glass ceiling was broken by a few, for a few, and the rest were left in a shower of shards. Legislative rights are available to all women, but it is only in more recent history that women of color and women who represent other types of minority statuses or intersectionality have achieved the same opportunities and successes as their white counterparts.

I often tell my students (and remind myself) that it is a fallacy to judge the actions of anyone without considering the historical context in which they lived. The same holds true for our baby boomers. The reality is that the slow rollout of women's rights and opportunities that impacted the move into midlife set the stage for how subsequent generations of women can experience their midlife transitions and do them differently than their mothers and grandmothers were able to.

Every generation of women experiences midlife in different ways. The leading edge of midlife women as of this writing are the Gen X women who are in their late forties through their sixties. In the middle is a microgeneration of Xennials who are sandwiched between Gen X and millennials, who share characteristics of both generations to some degree. And finally, millennials are beginning their sojourn into midlife in their unique manner. Most research on women's generational experiences of midlife centers on either Gen X or millennials; a defining characteristic of Gen X women's experiences is that they were the first to attain large-scale success in the professional world. Though some may tout this group as some of the "healthiest, wealthiest, and most active generation in history" (Falk, 2018); these women have also been classed as more perfectionistic and susceptible to burnout than their peers. Per author Ada Calhoun's (2020) qualitative book on Gen X women's experiences in midlife, women at this stage were fed the notion that they could do it all, be it all, and have it all, only to find that striving for "all" has left them depleted, exhausted, and realizing that such levels of achievement are unattainable and doesn't necessarily create happiness and fulfillment.

Millennials easing into their midlife years have experienced a major recession, recognizing that the ongoing wealth and prosperity of their early childhood isn't necessarily guaranteed. Indeed, this is a generation that has less money to spend than its Gen X counterparts due to the rising costs of living, which has outpaced their salaries more than previous generations (Hoffower & Kiersz, 2021). As a group, they tend to spend their money on experiences rather than things and are less likely to experience divorce than their other generational counterparts, because they are less likely to marry in the first place. Many women of this generation experience their midlife crises by feeling discontent and disconnected with their careers and work lives, which they may look to as their main mechanisms for personal fulfillment and find them sorely lacking (Miller, 2017).

What women of each of these generations have going for them is educational attainment: they have outpaced men within their generational cohorts. This can translate into more career opportunities and economic stability in the face of destabilizing events during their later lives. It also may imply that they are better educated than women of previous generations regarding available resources that can help them during life transitions, such as mental health care, financial literacy, and self-advocacy. Unifying factors for midlife women of any generation are challenges with coping with multiple simultaneous life stressors, such as breaking up a marriage or partnership, managing single life if they chose not to partner, death of parents, raising children, personal health issues, career challenges, and securing enough resources to meet household needs. With these issues also arises the existential crisis of personal fulfillment in the face of attending to others' interests and needs before their own. This can leave women in midlife feeling bereft and uncertain, wondering how they became stuck in what once may have seemed like the "right" path for them.

HOW DOES THIS PROBLEM REAR ITS HEAD?

Unhappiness takes many forms and can manifest in one's life as general malaise and low-level discomfort to more extreme behaviors such as addiction or severe mental illness. In this section, we explore the manifestations of problems that can occur and be exacerbated by life circumstances during midlife. You may see yourself or others in these examples. Keep an open mind; some of these experiences may resonate with you and some may not.

General malaise and existential angst is a common symptom across the lifespan, and it is completely appropriate to experience distress during times of transition (such as partnering) or uncertainty about life circumstances (changing jobs, moving). It becomes problematic when it progresses to a low-level constant in your life that you can't seem to shake, like a ten-pound weight that you carry with you all the time. Ten pounds isn't much—it doesn't feel heavy enough to mention and might be easy to ignore at times—but the metaphorical "weight" can prevent you from experiencing contentment in your daily life.

More intense experiences of unhappiness can include issues with relationships, feeling stuck in your job or career path, and consistently using sarcasm or gallows humor to cope. In my experience working with women in midlife and my own experiences with this life transition, what I've noticed is that women at this stage of life often begin to question some of the relationships that they have cultivated and maintained during their lives. Particularly, women begin to look at the time and energy that they have put into certain relationships and whether the energy is well spent. The cumulative effect of this type of reflection can be a culmination of unresolved anger and resentments that become a focal point for an individual's unhappiness. The big casualties of these reflections and inventories can be marriages/partnerships, work/career, and home life.

Let's start with the truth: being in a marriage or committed partnership is hard work. It starts with passion and fun, and it might be celebrated with a big fancy party. You are on a path to share your life with a person whom you love and who loves you back. That's the start of the fun part, and it takes work to keep it fun and find contentment in daily life. The unfun parts are the struggles: being broke, your partner's habits that make you nuts, family demands that you can't or don't want to meet, moving to a new place and establishing new ties, crying babies (and a partner who sleeps through it even though you've been up all night)—the list goes on. The sum of "unfun" and daily life without the buffer of positive experiences within the partnership can result in a long-term erosion of the relationship. The consequences of this erosion can create volatility in a partnership.

Feeling stuck in your job or career also can be a big sign of existential angst for a lot of reasons. It often forces us to ask the question, "What am I doing with my life?!" particularly when we consider how much time we spend working or engaging in the emotional labor of caring for our family and lives. According to the US Bureau of Labor Statistics (2023), the average woman spends approximately thirty-six hours a week on work and work-related tasks; this number includes part- and full-time workers. You may find yourself on either side of that spectrum: working a shorter number of hours at a formal job but spending a good deal of time on unpaid labor, or working longer hours, multiple jobs, and maintaining a household. Wherever you are on that spectrum, career in midlife can feel like being adrift, somewhere in the middle, with no changes in the foreseeable future. Career issues can be challenging because during midlife we have a great number of responsibilities that can impede us from making radical changes. Balancing responsibility with the need for fulfillment is an obstacle that many women face.

When we're stuck in the daily grind of work, we may choose to cope in other ways to manage our discontent. One of the ways is through using sarcasm and gallows humor. Don't get me wrong, using sarcasm can be a great way to cope, showing quick wit and cleverness. However, when sarcasm becomes the main way that you communicate, when it remains dark or negative, and when it is used to make fun *of* others instead of making fun *with* others, it quickly becomes toxic and destructive. A variation of this type of humor is gallows humor, which refers to humor that makes fun of life-threatening or frightening situations—such as work danger or traumas. One common American idiom is the phrase "going postal," which originates from the 1986 Edmond, Oklahoma, post office shooting, highly publicized as one of the first large-scale mass shootings at a workplace in the United States. Much like sarcasm, the use of this type of coping in microdoses can be useful and even a way for coworkers to bond over challenging situations. But when it becomes a part of the culture or ethos of one's approach to work and career, it sparks a downward spiral that can lead to unintended consequences, such as long-term unhappiness or potentially destructive coping mechanisms.

ROCK BOTTOM HAS A BASEMENT

Now you're thinking, *how much worse can this all get?* As many of us know, it can always get worse (see the gallows humor there?). In my experience as a counselor, people often exacerbate already challenging situations by using negative coping mechanisms to try to feel better. Coping mechanisms are what they sound like: ways to cope with difficult feelings and thoughts. Defining negative coping varies with the individual but relates to how they engage in the behavior. For example, many folks say that zoning out with a movie feels like a healthy escape. That's true, but when it becomes eight hours a day of zoning out to shows, social media, and so on, and it impedes other life activities, it's a problem.

The most common types of negative coping that I've seen in my clinical practice include alcohol and drug use, overspending/shopping, overeating/binge eating, and over-engagement with media and social media. Clients' stories about how these issues become problematic suggest a "creeping" type of problem that starts as healthy coping and, somewhere along the line, gradually creeps toward dysfunction. With any of the coping skills above, this is easily seen. For example, during the pandemic, alcohol sales and deliveries skyrocketed as people spent more time at home, were increasingly isolated, and social distancing and fear took their toll. What may have started as a fun way to play around with new cocktail recipes as a distraction became a way to numb oneself from the fearful reality of hearing news reports of death tolls from around the world. Although the pandemic is a very specific example, we see these impairments play out in our "return to normal" as women pick up the tasks of living. Working, caring for others, and trying to engage in their interests with more limited resources than before due to inflation in the global market, daily news about mass shootings, and world unrest are all stressors in women's lives that must be coped with in some way. Given our place in our collective history and the unrelenting demands on women's time and resources—especially in midlife, with so many simultaneous responsibilities—it's no wonder that engaging in more initially healthy coping skills is attractive.

An area in which I struggle is overeating and occasional binge eating in the face of stress. I recently spoke with a neighbor after returning from my vacation, and she commented that I looked like I'd lost weight. I joked with her that, of course I did—I hadn't been at work and needed to stress eat for the last few weeks. Our conversation lingered with me, and I kept mulling over how true it was. It's a running joke at my office that I need to keep stashes of chocolate around in case I'm particularly stressed and feel the need to indulge after a challenging meeting or interaction. Everyone knows—and even asks—*do you need chocolate?* I appreciate how attuned my colleagues are to me, and I confess that if my days didn't feel so rushed, I might try to walk off my feelings rather than eating them.

What makes me engage in this negative coping strategy? First, it's a habit. I got into the habit of using carbs as a coping mechanism earlier in my job and now I continue to use them. Second, it's quick. It takes very little effort to mindlessly unwrap candy to eat or to grab a bag of chips to munch on. Third, this habit is self-reinforcing. Eating things like chocolate or crunchy, salty snacks provides my brain with rushes of endorphins, the "painkiller" hormone I crave when I feel stressed or upset (Oliveira et al., 2020). Additionally, crunchy snacks provide a rush of dopamine, the "feel good" hormone that I want when I'm feeling sad or disappointed.

Unfortunately, self-reinforcing habits can be hard to break, and when the consequences seem somewhat minimal (weight flux), it is challenging to understand why one would change. But the longer the habit continues, the greater one's dependence on the coping mechanism, and the greater the consequences can become. In my case, stress eating led to cholesterol issues and related potential heart issues. My biggest problem was that I was still ignoring the underlying issue—my stress at work—and how I might make changes to cope with it differently. This resulted in a multiheaded health issue that grew much larger than it should have. I bet many of you can relate.

The slippery slope of creeping coping doesn't stop with the usual suspects of alcohol, drugs, and food. It can be found in any behavior that was once identified as healthy but that has become problematic enough for either you or others to notice. Social media use is one that I know many people struggle with. We use social media for several good purposes: for relevant information and entertainment, to market our businesses, and to keep up with people we care about. But how many of us have gone down the social media rabbit hole, realizing an hour later that we've spent way more time than we intended looking at videos of makeup tutorials, new dances, or funny memes or reels.

Social media can be a fun distraction, but when we're using it to avoid our lives or aren't even noticing that it's sucking up more of our lives than we realized, it's a problem. Comparing our lives to carefully curated photos and portrayals of others on social media has been shown to lead to issues with depression among social media users; social media overuse also contributes to loneliness, which has been deemed a public health epidemic (Meshi & Ellithorpe, 2021). Although not the sole reason for it, social media use also can lead individuals into greater spending habits due to influencing. We've all seen our favorite social media personality share with us the latest and greatest item through their feed, LTK app, or whatever other platform they're using to let us know what we're missing out on. If you remember your lessons in propaganda from school, you know that this type of influencing is not new or unique, but because marketing campaigns saturate the media, we are much more susceptible to being manipulated into believing that a certain dress, cream, or whatever will change our lives for the better.

It is highly unlikely that these products will change our lives in meaningful ways. But what these "investments" can do is become a drain on our finances. Some women in midlife may be experiencing a bit more spending power than they had in their early lives as they begin to see higher wages from years of working. One of the ways to celebrate these accomplishments is by rewarding oneself with extras or treats. In moderation this is fine, but if it becomes anything like my chocolate habit, it can be problematic, leading to financial shortfalls, debt, and arguments with partners about how money is being spent.

What all these coping skills have in common is that, if left unchecked, they can wreak havoc in your life. What starts as a fun or low-stakes way to shake off your stress has the potential to become something much greater. Part of the reason for this is that your brain needs to reach a certain threshold of stimulation to release the feel-good hormones you're seeking when you use these coping skills. Some release is easier to access (using drugs or alcohol), whereas other forms of release may take longer due to an increasingly higher threshold required to create the same reward. For example, individuals who are addicted to social media need to seek increased amounts of time and exposure to the stimulus to achieve the same pleasure from it (Zivnuska et al., 2019). So you may have initially enjoyed fifteen minutes scrolling on Instagram or watching YouTube, whereas now you find yourself checking your feed at various points throughout the day, sometimes for an hour or more at a time. Because you've engaged with social media for prolonged periods, you now need to spend more time to get the same reward that you once achieved with a fifteen-minute scroll. The "need" to engage becomes both longer and more frequent until it can become intrusive to your life. Have you ever seen families who are out to dinner, and everyone is staring at their phones? One of the reasons could be that everyone is trying to get their "fix." I know—I'm telling you things that you already know and have read about . . . which are all true and can cause lasting effects on both how you feel about yourself and how others perceive you.

PERMISSION TO TAKE A MENTAL HEALTH DAY—OR MONTH

Finally, another manifestation of feeling unhappy or stuck in midlife can be the onset of anxiety and depression. This is not a chicken-and-egg argument (which came first, midlife or mental health issues?). First, it is insulting because, since the dawn of psychoanalysis (thanks, Freud) and way before, women have been subjected to all manner of stigma based on their sex, gender identity, and the societal role that is placed upon them by those in power. No matter where you are in life, historically, being a female has been synonymous with labels such as "hysteria." Second, being aware of and actively seeking treatment for mental health issues is universally healthy and appropriate for all people; not everyone has equal access to mental health treatment. There are many reasons that folks don't have access to this medical necessity from lack of insurance or funds to denial of problems, stigma, or shame.

Why might mental health issues present themselves in midlife differently than during other phases of life? In my practice, I have seen that midlife is the point at which people not only take a serious inventory of what they have done with their lives to date, but they also realize that some of the expectations that they have of themselves or that others have for them are not realistic or desirable. Sometimes, even in the face of these issues, women try to continue their course, staying in the same dysfunctional relationships, jobs, churches, and so on because they feel that the situation will get better and/or the thought of changing their lives is more frightening than staying the same. When this happens, often there is an incongruence between how a woman thinks, feels, and behaves. At its core, incongruence can be thought of as a conflict between one's aspirational values and the compromises one makes in the course of living their life. Over time, living in a state of incongruence between thoughts, feelings, and behaviors can become exhausting. Left unchecked, it is toxic and can take a toll on your mental health.

For a low-stakes example, imagine you're in the grocery store and you see an acquaintance that you don't like. For some reason, this individual did something to you that still makes you angry. You see them first and, in your head, you think, "Ugh! It's them! They're awful!" As you keep walking, you feel your body tense, you start to feel angry just thinking about whatever it was that this person did, and you continue walking toward the orange juice, which is going to take you right past them. You don't have the option to abandon the cart, so you keep walking. What do you do? You could ignore them, but they are a social acquaintance, and you do see each other around town. Instead, you smile and say, "Hey there, how are you doing?" and keep walking.

This is an example of incongruence. Your thoughts and feelings were aligned, but your behavior belied those thoughts and feelings, and you were pleasant. This is a harmless example, as most people would not be overtly rude to someone they don't like when they happen to bump into them in the grocery store. But if your life is about consistently denying your thoughts, emotions, and behaviors, then it is a recipe for serious mental anguish. Consistently sublimating or denying your real experience of the world in favor of someone else's point of view or to keep the peace is not only unhealthy but also dangerous to your psyche. It is the denial of who you are—the values, beliefs, and boundaries that make up your internal sense of self—and will erode the essence of yourself. Left to continue, it can also lead to depression and/or anxiety, if not more serious issues.

Let me be clear that for many people, depression, anxiety, and other mental health issues are biological, such as chemical imbalance. When this occurs, it is important to seek treatment to help with imbalances; it is equally important to realize that medical intervention is only one part of staying well. Other components of staying well and maintaining mental health include living within your truth, congruently, and staying consistent in how you think, feel, and behave. What women tend to find is that they have managed (or ignored) these issues well until the cumulative effects of life stressors, incongruence, and negative coping mechanisms take their toll, and then their experiences of depression, anxiety, or other identified mental health issues worsen to the point that they must be addressed.

HOW DID WE GET HERE?

The question for many women at this stage is, "How did I get here?" They look at their lives and find themselves bewildered by all the things that they are doing by rote, without taking the time to consider if perhaps they need to do things a different way. There are many answers to this question, which range from "it's what I've always done/it's what my friends/family/others do" to "I'm not sure how to live my life any differently than how I am right now." Here's the thing that I admire most about women: they are resourceful and resilient. If you have picked up this book while you are feeling stuck and you're trying to figure out a solution, it means that you have the motivation to get unstuck and move forward. And looking at what got you here is important so that you can be vigilant when you find yourself stuck at future points in your life.

The most common reason that women tell me they feel stuck in their lives is their response to social or family messages that telegraph to them what their roles "should" be. Let's talk about "should." In the world of psychotherapy, and according to the theorist Albert Ellis, using the word "should" belongs to the world of irrational beliefs (Sharf, 2012, p. 336). An irrational belief defies logic, doesn't conform to our life experiences or wishes, and adheres to a set of internalized principles that doesn't serve us. Perfectionism is an example of an irrational belief that rears up especially hard during holidays. Ladies, how many of us have said, "I should make sure that everything in the house is picture-perfect because that is how my family will have a magical holiday season akin to those portrayed in all of those lovely and unrealistic holiday movies"? How many of us have run ourselves ragged to make sure that everything looks a certain way or have gone to extraordinary lengths to ensure that everything is "perfect" on a given holiday only to be exhausted, snappish, and resentful during the actual event because although it looked good, we were too tired to enjoy it? (Raises hand here.)

Special occasions aside, in our everyday lives, "should" and irrational beliefs are consistent companions that can prevent us from living our most refined lives within our values. Instead, they keep us in layers of busyness that distract us from our true purpose. "Should" can influence how we take care of our bodies and souls, nurture our loved ones, care for our homes, engage in our work, and interact with our communities. The purpose of this book is to consider multiple factors of wellness and the ways in which we are living that don't align with our core values. Going a step further, we must examine the ways in which we are stuck and move toward living in the values that serve us in this stage of our lives.

THE POWER OF FAMILY

I had coffee with one of my students and during our conversation, she expressed to me that she was pursuing a new religious path that was very different from the one that she grew up with. After a great deal of soul-searching and reflection, she realized that the religious values that she was raised with were contributing to internalized messages of shame and self-hatred. These negative schemas manifested themselves in her anxiety, her experience of an eating disorder, and her inability to safely maintain relationship boundaries with those closest to her. I admire her strength and fortitude; she is staying true to her belief that religion is a practice that brings a great deal of value to her life, and she is pursuing her religious and spiritual life away from her upbringing and her family's traditions, which was not an easy decision. This student is forging a path that is like my readers, casting out to see if there is a new path that serves them differently, perhaps better than the path they are on.

My student was given religious instruction and indoctrination early in her life from birth. These cultural expectations were transmitted through rituals, family expectations, and kinship ties to her community. There are so many things that we do without thinking about them: our spiritual practices, what we eat (or don't eat) for breakfast, the type of media that we consume, and so on. We often do these things out of habit, due to external expectations from others, or because they may be easy or the path of least resistance. Engaging in values, boundaries, and beliefs that no longer serve us is how we can become stuck.

Social messages are particularly important and can come from our community, peers, religious/spiritual organizations, media, and other places of influence. Social messages aren't social media or social media platforms, although social messaging can be conveyed through these mechanisms. A social message is an idea or value that is conveyed by a community regarding expectations for thoughts, behaviors, or feelings. In sociological terms, *norms* are a model that convey acceptable behaviors; *mores* are more fixed and express the expectations for subsets of groups (https://sociologydictionary.org/). For example, a social message may convey a norm that it's good for one's mental health to take time for self-care, but the mores may convey that a mother's self-care should come only after her children's needs are met.

We are inundated with social messages from the time that we're born (and even before if you think of the pink and blue paradigm) about what is expected of us based on who we are in society, and "society" likes stability or homeostasis. This means that when you try to do something different than the established norms or mores, it can be quite shocking, and you may receive pushback from others. The family serves as one of the most powerful organizations for transmitting messages regarding expectations, and working to stay in the family system is one of the most powerful reasons that individuals allow themselves to remain stuck in patterns that do not serve them. We will sacrifice a lot to maintain our family ties, including ourselves.

Family messages and expectations for behaviors are so powerful, and we don't tend to question them because the people who are related to us are supposed to love us and have our best interests at heart. I would like to believe that is true, and I think very often it is. There are individuals who are reading this who come from very challenging families of origin and have had to sever family ties to protect themselves from damage. There also may be those who are in toxic or problematic families who are not able to minimize exposure for a variety of reasons. My hope for all my readers is that you have found people in your lives, either family or family by choice, who are invested in your growth and well-being as an individual. That said, any family member who sends you messages about expectations for how you act has a major disadvantage: they don't live in your skin. How can someone who doesn't have your unique constellation of experiences know the intricacies of what you need to live in a meaningful way at this stage of your life?

When I teach the family counseling course at my university, I like to remind my students that if they see a family with five members, then they have to account for five different perspectives when taking a history. Even children raised in the same sibling set have different experiences of a given event and know different versions of their parents based on how their parents related to them as people. There is a saying that your family knows how to push your buttons because they're the ones who installed them, and to some degree that is true. The messages that you received as a child and into adulthood from your family about who you are and the place that you hold within the family can be a powerful reinforcement for the roles that you play in that system and the outside world. For example, who has met the firstborn, high-achieving sibling who overfunctions and takes care of everyone's needs before trouble starts? Who has met the middle child who goes with the flow and seldom demands much because they may not have gotten their way too often? These early experiences can create a template for who we become, but it is ultimately up to us to continue those patterns once we have emerged from our first families and become the adults we wish to be.

Other important family messages that can keep us stuck may be trauma, abuse, or attachment that has occurred during earlier phases in our lives. As children and adults, we internalize messages that we receive that give us pieces of information about ourselves and the world that make up our worldview. These messages can be driven by our environment. For example, the girl who grows up in a house where she was sexually abused may be perceived as putting herself into dangerous sexual situations as an adult. But if her earlier experiences were that her boundaries around her sexuality were violated, why would she believe that they could be respected when she became an adult, rather than consistently overruled? Another extreme example of this phenomenon is the woman who is so guarded about her personal safety that she is unable to engage in sexual or intimate relationships because she does not trust that her values will be honored, so it is better to remain alone or in a relationship where she can perceive that she has control.

These early traumas are one example, but traumas can happen later in life as well. Imagine a woman whose partner leaves her and who is unable to support herself and her family on her income. Resource insecurity, such as food, housing, healthcare, and childcare are real traumas that many women must push aside and move through to keep their families functioning. But these experiences are lasting traumas that can impact and affect a woman's future relationship with her children, family, future partners, and money.

Some of the most powerful messages that we receive come from ourselves. These are the internalized scripts that create limits for us that can be more powerful than any other external force. This is the voice from our conscience from which we hear our self-doubts, our worst criticism of ourselves, and from which we perpetuate internalized messages of shame and fear that can keep us stuck. In my experience as a counselor and as a human, these are the messages that tell us we're not good enough or smart enough to take a certain risk, that we're not worthy of being loved or cared for, that to be "good," we must put others first and ourselves last—always and without consideration for what we may need. Sometimes the narrative is more innocuous; maybe it's the voice that says, "I have so much, what could I possibly have to complain about?" It is the voice that tells you that you should be satisfied with what you have, even when it feels like a form of complacency. This is the voice of precontemplative change, which tells you all the ways you could change yet also gives you all the excuses as to why you can't change (Prochaska & Norcross, 2001). But you know—you know in your heart and your soul—that you are not happy, that you are not living within your values, and that this yearning can be satisfied only if you strive toward something different, toward change.

CHANGE IS SCARY

The problem is that the old ways of being and the things that we valued once in our lives no longer serve us. There isn't a place to lay blame; it is simply that, as we evolve, what we need as midlife adults evolves. And this is never truer than in midlife when we have the wisdom of our experiences coupled with a healthy respect for the fact that our time on this planet is finite. These insights are compounded, given that women face unique experiences in midlife due to our biology, gendered socialization, cultural expectations and restraints, and our specific time in history. As we begin to cast about because we feel a sense of discontent, what we realize is that we are not feeling fulfilled in some way. This can be an indication that we need to evaluate our values to see if they are still working for us or if they need to be reexamined or revised to align with who we are at this stage of our lives. When we align with our true values, we tend to be motivated to move toward them and sustain habits to maintain and live our values in meaningful ways.

Our motivations are what keep us moving every day; even negative motivations can keep us moving forward. My stress binge eating is an example of a negative motivation; I engaged in a self-soothing behavior that didn't align with my health values, and it cost me an aspect of my health that I had to work to get back. My motivation for self-soothing was stronger than my value for healthy coping, which meant that I needed to take an internal inventory of how I was functioning and which I valued more: my overall health or my need to engage in unhealthy coping. It took time to reorient myself to coping strategies that aligned with my values around health. It also took refining my boundaries with myself, others, and my work. In this way, many of us face the ultimate problem of being out of touch with our internal motivation, and we need to refine our values so we can find our motivation.

This isn't to say that the values, beliefs, and boundaries we ascribe to aren't good; many times they are. However, if we aren't examining how they align with our lives in midlife, if we aren't truly living our lives within these values, or if these values need to be revised to fit the circumstances that we find ourselves in, then we may be feeling the misalignment in our lives. Our task in this book is to look at the facets of wellness that we have control over, assess our values in these areas, revise and refine them for the women we are today, and begin living the best version of our lives at this stage. We will let go of the old values, beliefs, and boundaries that don't serve us and engage in a voyage of self-examination and evolution to move forward in this phase. This book will help by guiding you through a personal assessment of global wellness that align with the chapters of this book and then lead you through each facet by chapter, giving you some education and reflective exercises that will jump-start your self-discovery journey. Let's get started.

CHAPTER TWO

REDEFINING WELLNESS

I was speaking with one of my clients and she said something that resonated with me: in the summer of 2023 it felt as though many of us were relaxing our jaws, releasing the tension that built up during the last few years with the pandemic and the turmoil that has ensued due to world unrest. I believe this accurately describes how many of us are feeling globally. I also think that when we are in our midlife years, our responsibilities are endless, regardless of the additional challenges we've dealt with since 2020. Our personal, day-to-day stressors combined with world stressors have created a perfect storm of tension, fear, and fatigue that may be clouding our ability to live well and fully.

So, as we start this chapter, please begin by taking a deep breath. Allow yourself to notice where your breath goes as it moves into your body. Does it stop at the top of your chest, or does it go deeper into your lungs, allowing your ribcage to expand? Maybe you want to consider reclining so that you can breathe more deeply and encourage the breath down into your stomach, allowing it to expand. Imagine a baby breathing. They breathe with their whole torso, and they breathe all the way into their stomachs, allowing their diaphragm to expand and contract. Allow yourself the time and space to take at least ten deep breaths. You can do this in silence or with sound; try to find a space where you feel safe and can relax. You might want to close or soften your eyes so that you can pay attention to how the breath moves in and out of your body. As you continue to breathe, take the opportunity to unhinge your jaw, maybe also massaging the muscles in your jaw area to help loosen them up. Continue breathing and notice the difference in your body after you've completed these exercises.

How do you feel? Most individuals report feeling calmer when they've completed this exercise. Science holds with that assessment. When we slow down our breath and relax our muscles, we regulate our nervous system. Our breathing impacts the vagus nerve, which regulates our sympathetic nervous system, also known as the "fight, flight, or freeze" part of the brain. Slow breathing is one way that we can engage the parasympathetic nervous system, which controls the "rest and digest" part of our brains, allowing us to relax and rest. Have you ever noticed that when you are "elevated" in some way (with a higher heart rate, rapid breathing, and/or tense muscles) you may make decisions that are not as well thought out as they would be if you were relaxed and able to reflect? That's the difference between decision making when you're experiencing stress (sympathetic nervous system) rather than when you're calm (parasympathetic nervous system).

Now that you're in a calmer state, let's move into assessing your current wellness. I want to reinforce that this book and the exercises contained therein are private spaces that neither I nor your friends and family will see. Relax. I hope that you're reading this book to learn and that you're going to also have some fun and gain some insights about yourself to further refine how you are in the world. You might learn some things that you want to change, and you are going to find some things you're doing pretty well. Keep this in mind as we move forward on this journey of self-discovery, evolution, and refinement.

HOW SATISFIED ARE YOU WITH YOUR OVERALL WELLNESS?

The Global Assessment of Functioning (GAF) Scale is a measure that was once used to help assess individuals' psychological, social, and occupational functionality on a continuum of health and illness using a 100-point scale. You've seen similar types of scaling at doctor's offices for pain, such as using a 1–10 scale to determine levels of pain. In this section, I've adapted these ideas to create a scale that I call a global wellness assessment. Using it, you can rank your perception of your wellness based on scaling questions that will help you to focus on the areas of wellness discussed in this book. Several things to keep in mind: (1) Lower numbers indicate a lower level of satisfaction compared to higher numbers. (2) What one number means to you isn't the same as what it means to someone else, so I ask you to take an extra step and define what your numbers mean to you. (3) Your satisfaction will vary among the wellness categories, which is to be expected. (4) Consider what it means for you to be satisfied with a particular number. Although this process is focused on growth, that shouldn't negate your satisfaction with a particular aspect of your wellness. Completing an assessment and being happy about a particular benchmark in your wellness is something to be celebrated. There is something very important about not continually striving toward all things and in relaxing and resting with the achievements that you've made.

GLOBAL ASSESSMENT OF WELLNESS EXERCISE

Directions: Assess your overall health and wellness based on the definitions and numbers below. Note that lower numbers indicate a lower level of satisfaction as compared to higher numbers. Choose a number (1–10) that best reflects your satisfaction (during the last six months) with this indicator of wellness.

Mental health: Satisfaction with your overall emotional, psychological, and social well-being

1   5   10

Physical health: Satisfaction includes your ability to recover from illness and the state of your physical body and its operations (base your score on things that you can control as well as those you cannot)

1   5   10

Appearance: Satisfaction in accepting your body and holding a favorable opinion of it, internalizing your opinion about beauty standards rather than stereotypical or cultural standards of beauty

1   5   10

Intimate relationships: Satisfaction with relationships in which both parties are mutually responsive to one another's needs during both painful and happier times of life

1   5   10

CHAPTER TWO

Social health: Satisfaction with relationships and connections within one's community; having a sense of belonging to groups, which may include friends, family, and other important groups

1   5   10

Vocational/career health: Satisfaction with and enrichment from one's work; ideally, work that aligns with your skills and values and that provides a sense of fulfillment ("work" includes paid work and volunteer positions)

1   5   10

Leisure health: Satisfaction with the activities that you do on a voluntary, non-work-related basis

1   5   10

Spiritual health: Satisfaction with your connection to a higher power or connection with something that is beyond the self (such as nature or a specific deity)

1   5   10

For each of these dimensions of personal wellness functioning, complete the following:

1. Select your score for each of the dimensions from 1–10.
2. Create a definition for each number; for example, what does a 4 on your social health score mean to you?
3. What does your score tell you about what you are doing in this facet of wellness? What does your score tell you about what you may not be doing in this facet of wellness?

Mental health score

    Definition of score: _____

    What this score means to me: _____

Physical health score

    Definition of score: _____

    What this score means to me: _____

Appearance score

    Definition of score: _____

    What this score means to me: _____

Intimate relationships score

    Definition of score: _____

    What this score means to me: _____

Social health score

    Definition of score: _____

    What this score means to me: _____

Vocational/career health score

    Definition of score: _____

    What this score means to me: _____

Leisure health score

    Definition of score: _____

    What this score means to me: _____

Spiritual health score

    Definition of score: _____

    What this score means to me: _____

Establishing a Baseline

As you look at your scores, definitions, and the meanings that you attach to your scores, what do you observe? The purpose of this exercise is to determine where you are in your life and establish a baseline so that you can modulate different facets of your wellness, which is the work of this book. What I often hear from women is that they are not where they want to be in their wellness and their development, and they offer a lot of good reasons for why they aren't where they want to be. Many of those reasons are forces outside of them, including family responsibilities, work expectations, conflicting commitments, and the list goes on. However, if we want to be the most refined version of ourselves—living and embodying the wisdom of who we are and how we can best function in our lives—we also must be very truthful with ourselves about when we are ceding responsibility for our wellness to these external forces rather than taking responsibility for living our best lives.

This book will help you to tailor your values, boundaries, and beliefs for the woman you are: a powerful woman moving into a new phase of her life with the wisdom to know that evolution is healthy, possible, and necessary. Many women look outside of themselves for cues about how they "should" be; it's very similar to what we all did during our adolescent years. We looked to our peers to help us to normalize and figure out what we were supposed to value and do. We tend to do the same thing throughout our lifespan to some degree, but as we age we ultimately realize that no one is living our exact life with the same constellation of situations that we experience. As stated by Orson Welles, "We're born alone, we live alone, we die alone," and although that may seem a bit bleak, it is true that no one else is rattling around in our heads but us. We seek connections to feel less alone, but no one else can live this life that we've been given, so we need to move forward to define and refine our values, boundaries, and beliefs and live within them in order to be true to ourselves.

A DEEPER LOOK AT VALUES, BOUNDARIES, AND BELIEFS

Values

According to Merriam-Webster, *value* (noun) has eight definitions, but the one most relevant to this discussion is "something (such as principle or quality) intrinsically valuable or desirable." The natural question to ask is, *what do you value?* What principles hold meaning for you and are desirable for you to hold on to? When we're younger, we're taught the values of our parents, and we tend to go in one of two directions: we adopt them as our own or we reject them as not useful in our lives. For example, as children, we say to our mothers, "When I have kids, I'm never going to make them . . ." and we follow through. Or, through our own experiences, we realize that our mothers are human and have some insights that we don't. (Though I still get irritated when I realize my mother was right about so many things.)

Adolescence is the developmental time in life when we formulate our initial values (both retaining and rejecting the values that we learned in childhood) and begin building our young adult lives based on those values. Here's the thing that no one explicitly says: *we're not done developing our values at the age of twenty-five.* In your head, you know this, but when was the last time you examined your values? Also, when was the last time you asked yourself whether you are living within the values that are important to you? Some of them, yes, but some of them, maybe not.

We all have strongly held values and beliefs that align with the spheres of wellness discussed in the subsequent chapters of this book. These values can encompass our thoughts about our spiritual or religious lives and belief systems, how we eat, who our friends are, how we present ourselves to the world, and the list goes on. In the preface, we saw how Casey was attempting to live within values that no longer served her. In that example, Casey prized work and novelty above other values, which served her for a period, but she found that she changed. Although work and novelty are still values for her, they are no longer her highest priority.

Growing up in the South, the value of respect was expected by most adults. I did not grow up in a house with traditional Southerners, but I did go to school and had to learn about adults' expectations regarding respect. I learned the response of "Yes, ma'am" and "Yes, sir" very quickly. This is also a good example of how values can be very culturally encapsulated. When I visited my mother's family in the western United States, they were confused by my formality, which probably did sound funny from a six-year-old. Over time, I learned to code-switch, understanding my audience and what was expected from one adult versus another. But the importance of respect was impressed upon me at an early age. Because it was culturally important and expected, showing respect to adults and elders through my actions and using certain language, such as *ma'am* and *sir*, are values that I still carry with me, though not to the same degree. I still think that it is important to be respectful to others, but I also have a better understanding that individuals need to earn my respect rather than be given it freely.

This is just one example of values and how they evolve. Realizing that my respect needed to be earned rather than freely given to someone due to expectation or status evolved slowly over time. Climbing the ranks of higher education as both a graduate student and faculty member, it is expected to show a level of deference to those with more degrees and experience than you. I will also say that there are some real jerks in higher education, although there are jerks everywhere. The realization that not everyone garnered equal respect from me (although they thought they deserved it) was a slow lesson for me. That probably sounds extremely naive to my readers, and I think it is likely a result of starting my education and academic career at a relatively young age compared to others. I think it also has to do with my gendered experiences of living and working in the South, where gender role expectations have not changed as quickly as in other parts of the country.

I hope that after reading my example about the value of respect you can think of some of your own values that have evolved, perhaps unconsciously. The purpose of this section is to allow you to review a set of values that are important to you and to consider how you think about them now as opposed to how you may have thought about them in the past. There is something very liberating about reflecting on how you thought about certain values in the past and acknowledging that the way that you hold those values now is different and congruent with the person who you are today. Even as I write this section and think about the value of respect, I smile to myself because I realize that my definition of respect has expanded beyond the definition I was handed as a youngster and encompasses not just people, but the world around me. How can I be respectful of my own time and others' time? How can I be respectful to strangers in my town? How can I be respectful of another culture or group when I am traveling abroad? When I take the time to reflect on this value, I realize that I still hold it as important. However, my definition of respect is much broader and my boundaries for individuals to maintain my respect are far stronger than they used to be.

VALUES SORT EXERCISE

Let's move forward in this section by completing a values sort, which is a brief exercise that asks you to look at a list of values and circle the ones that are most important to you. It doesn't mean that the values that aren't selected are unimportant; it simply means that we must make decisions about our priorities and work within those priorities. As you review this list, consider where you are at this point in your life. Midlife is a fine balance of owning your experiences, moving forward with the wisdom of your past experiences, and recognizing the finite time you have to live your life. As you look at this list, consider what your top values are now. It might be helpful to create a list of your top values from the past and how these have changed over time.

Listed below are 120 values presented in alphabetical order. Read through them when you have time to reflect on how these words resonate with you. You'll notice that some words may seem very similar, but in fact have different meanings and nuances. Choose the top ten values that are the most meaningful to you in this phase of your life. One way to think about which values are important to you is to recall a time you were angry because a value was violated; this is a great way to dig deep and identify what matters to you.

Abundance	Awareness	Confidence
Acceptance	Balance	Conformity
Accountability	Beauty	Cooperation
Achievement	Bravery	Courage
Adaptability	Calmness	Creativity
Adventure	Caring	Curiosity
Affection	Change	Decisiveness
Alone time	Clarity	Dedication
Altruism	Cleanliness	Dependability
Appreciation	Cleverness	Diversity
Artistry	Community	Efficiency
Autonomy	Compassion	Empathy

Encouragement
Entertainment
Enthusiasm
Equal relationship
Exploration
Fairness
Faith
Fame
Family
Fidelity
Financial security
Forgiveness
Freedom
Friendship
Generosity
Gratitude
Happiness
Harmony
Honesty
Honor
Hope
Humility
Humor
Imagination
Independence
Influence
Innovation
Integrity
Intimacy
Intuition
Joy/fun
Justice
Kindness
Knowledge
Leisure
Listening
Loyalty
Modesty
Nonconformity
Nonviolence
Open-mindedness
Optimism
Organization
Passion
Patience
Persistence
Personal development
Positive attitude
Power
Professionalism
Prosperity
Quality
Quality time
Reciprocity
Reliability
Religion
Resourcefulness
Respect
Responsibility
Romance
Self-love
Self-motivation
Self-preservation
Selflessness
Sincerity
Social justice
Spirituality
Spontaneity
Stability
Strength
Success
Sustainability
Thoughtfulness
Timeliness
Tolerance
Tradition
Transparency
Travel
Trust
Understanding
Vivaciousness
Wealth
Wellness
Wisdom

REFLECTION QUESTIONS

- What made these values most important to you at this stage of your life?
- How are you living these values in your daily life? (How do you think, feel, and behave in alignment with these values?)
- How are you not living these values in your daily life? (How do you not think, feel, and behave in alignment with these values?)
- If there is a misalignment between your values and your thoughts, feelings, and behaviors, what might need to shift?
- How do your selected values differ from what you may have valued at a different stage of life?
- What does this value shift tell you about yourself?

Knowing and prioritizing your values can have a positive impact on the next concepts we discuss, which are beliefs/motivations and boundaries. Living within your values means that you are committed to them; this includes thinking, feeling, and acting in ways that align with your values. In the next section, we explore how your belief in your values is an important aspect of maintaining motivation to act and move toward what you value. Then we explore how maintaining boundaries can help you to align with your values. Boundaries that are driven by your values can help you to refine your daily life, shaking off things that don't align with your values and may not be serving you during this phase of your life.

Beliefs

Belief (noun) has three definitions and the one we'll use for our purposes is "a state or habit of mind in which trust or confidence is placed in some person or thing." The part of this definition that I love is "habit of mind." Isn't this what so many of us are subject to do, lapsing into habits without fully thinking through *why* we do the things that we do? And these beliefs can range from the serious to the silly, depending on the subject. I really believe that spaghetti is better when I put the sauce on top of the noodles and mix them together myself. I live with someone who believes that spaghetti is better when the sauce and noodles are mixed before serving. The mild irritation I feel when serving myself mixed sauce and noodles is both ridiculous and the result of a habit of mind. Habits can be self-limiting and result in rigid thinking about how we can conduct our lives; in essence, these are walls that we build around ourselves that box us into rigid functioning and ultimately contribute to our belief systems. When we become aware that these walls are self-imposed and can be broken down, we allow ourselves the freedom to think creatively and examine our beliefs in new ways to determine if they still serve us.

By the same token, habits and beliefs also can be very powerful in helping us maintain certain behaviors without having to think too hard about doing them. For example, brushing our teeth in the morning isn't something we have to think about. We do it because we believe oral health is important and cultivate a habit that reinforces the behavior. In this case, we've enforced the habit to the point that if we don't do it, we might feel uncomfortable. Harnessing the power of beliefs and habits is a useful tool in our quest to live our most refined lives, but we must examine these to ensure that our beliefs and the resulting habits are aligned with our values and truly benefit us at this stage of our lives.

A recent example of the power of beliefs came from popular culture when Jennifer Aniston revealed that she changed her workout regime because her old habits resulted in several serious injuries that compounded over time. In her story, she discussed her belief that if she wasn't completing forty-five minutes of high-impact cardio per day, then she wasn't working out. For some people, the cumulative effect of daily high-impact workouts can cause damage to joints and make it challenging for muscles to repair after hard use, and repeated impact can cause undue stress to the skeletal structure. In Ms. Aniston's example, she spent years doing the same types of workouts with similar resulting injuries until a physical therapist intervened, using as a visual aid a doll with kinetic tape on it to illustrate the extent of her bodily injuries due to her adherence to this punishing workout habit.

What Jennifer Aniston needed to reexamine was her beliefs about exercise and her value of physical wellness. Likely she is very dedicated to her physical health, but her belief that to achieve and maintain it she needed to engage in high-impact workouts was damaging her body.

With the help of a professional, she gained insight that her belief about physical health was ultimately damaging, and perhaps she realized that the cumulative effects of her injuries may not result in a healthy body as she aged into her middle and later adult years. The result of this insight was the infusion of *flexibility* into her belief: recognition that there are multiple avenues toward optimal physical health and that dogmatic adherence to one path (high-impact cardio) would not benefit her in the next phases of her life. Maybe there had been past consequences she had ignored.

Flexibility is not a word you often hear in relation to beliefs, but I want you to consider how flexibility may be beneficial to you. As you reflect on your beliefs based on the values that you circled on the values sort, how might you be rigid and dogmatic in how you adhere to your beliefs around these values? How might you be more flexible and give yourself more latitude in your beliefs? In the earlier example, Ms. Aniston's ability to become more flexible in her beliefs about physical exercise gave her greater mental and emotional freedom to broaden her definition of physical health, which may have resulted in a wider variety of physical activities and helped her to appreciate the benefits of rest and lower impact activities as part of her health habits. Considering how you might broaden your view of a particular belief and be more flexible in how you express it in your life can be an interesting personal exercise.

A counterpoint to becoming more flexible is thinking about the boundaries that govern how you live within your values and beliefs. In the next section, we consider the types of boundaries that you may have and examine how boundaries are imperative to living your most refined life.

Boundaries

Boundaries (noun) are defined as "something that indicates or fixes a limit or extent." I have found that many boundaries are drawn in the sand rather than concrete. What I mean is that although some personal boundaries may be more fixed—such as an individual's belief about their religious or spiritual life—other boundaries may be subject to "drift" and change or be manipulated over time. For example, in a conversation with my cousin the other day, she talked about how she didn't feel well at work and told her boss that she may need to go home. She was certain she was sick and adamant that she needed to get home and rest. Her boss requested that she stay until the end of the day since there was an important meeting scheduled. My cousin agreed and stayed through the meeting only to go home and find out she had COVID. Not only was she sick, but she also may have infected her coworkers. A lot of boundaries come into play here for both my cousin and her boss, such as those around personal health, following rules at work, respect for other individuals' boundaries, considering the welfare of others, and so on. With this example, one of the most challenging issues is the power differential between an employee and their supervisor and how that impacted how the situation played out.

Boundaries that are harder to define or that are situationally dependent (aka "drawn in the sand") are challenging because they change. Individuals are expected to evolve and change over time, as are boundaries, but when we don't have a clear notion about our boundaries and how they align with our values and beliefs, then it becomes challenging for us to function optimally, and we may find ourselves in situations that don't serve us. A prime example of this is saying yes to a lot of different activities, opportunities, and tasks in our lives (this can also extend to saying yes on behalf of partners, children, etc.). When we say "Yes!" to all the opportunities that come our way, we may find that we are busier than we want to be. Our new activities detract from our core values when they take us away from focusing energy on the people and things that are most important to us.

Another important insight about boundaries is that sometimes we don't know that one has been pushed beyond its limit until it occurs. Many of us can think back to a time when we found ourselves in a situation with another person who pushed the limits of a personal boundary. Pushing past the limits of a boundary is sometimes called a boundary violation; a personal reaction to a boundary violation is often an emotional response such as frustration or anger. When a boundary violation occurs with a value that is clearly defined, it is easier to understand the emotional reaction we experience. When the boundary violation occurs in relation to a less well-defined boundary, the emotional reaction may still be frustration or anger, but pinpointing the "why" behind the emotion is more challenging. Often these situations leave us feeling confused and it may take time to reflect and determine the reasons behind our turmoil.

A recent example occurred in my work life. I was invited to participate on an interdisciplinary team to set up a working clinic on an area of campus. I was excited to work with the team because I'm always thrilled to be a part of building something that can help others. After several disjointed meetings with a lack of clear direction, I came to realize that although I had been invited to be on this team, my perception was that my thoughts and ideas about the project were not taken into consideration. Additionally, when I offered information about the limits of the project, which was well within my expertise, it was dismissed as unimportant. Now don't get me wrong, you're reading this example and thinking, "This chick got her ego bruised and now she's picking up her toys and going home."

Well, I'm human and I do struggle with my ego, so I certainly reflected on feeling dismissed. What I also reflected on is that I do value being respected, both my knowledge level (for which I have worked more than twenty years to obtain) as well as my time. When I say yes to one project, I am saying no to something else that I value. What I wasn't aware of until it occurred was that this interdisciplinary project team did not value my time and contributions, and that time spent on building the clinic project was taking time away from writing this book. I value respect, and my belief about respect is that it should be mutual, coming from both parties. I was angry because I felt that my time was being wasted with a team that didn't value my input or respect my time and commitment. Ultimately the choice to continue belonged to me, which is freeing, because although I believe in following through on my commitments, if the commitment isn't productive or if my contributions to the commitment are not needed, then I must allow myself to choose to stop engaging in it. Is this always possible? Absolutely not.

In this case, it was possible, and I am now writing this paragraph after refining my boundaries around respecting my time and my beliefs and expectations for how others should respect my time. My most important insight in this situation was ensuring that my decisions align with my goals and commitments when I have the autonomy to choose how I spend my time. The importance of this lesson lies in *remembering* it and *putting it into practice* when future opportunities arise. When I make future commitments, I must ask myself: How is joining this project respecting my own time and current commitments? How do I expect to be treated by others if I commit to this project? How will I also engage in respecting others committed to this project? If I later discover that this commitment is not something that I can follow through on due to issues regarding respect and time, how will I handle the situation?

Have you ever seen a yard with spray paint at the edges to mark the electric, gas, or water lines? The paint marks the boundaries to make it safe to engage in home projects. After time, grass grows and the lines become faint and likely wash away or are cut away after mowing. Our boundaries can be like that: we can define them but over time they fade and we forget where the lines were drawn. When that occurs, it is important to take a personal inventory to redraw the lines for ourselves and others. Unlike lines buried in a yard, our lines can shift and evolve; this is to be expected. But consistent inventories to clarify where the lines are drawn can save us a lot of heartache, or in the case of construction, broken water lines and a flood of emotions.

So what does it mean to have healthy boundaries? The word *boundary*, in therapeutic terms, refers to a set of rules or guidelines that an individual creates that indicates how other people should behave around them or treat them. Boundaries are subjective and based on an individual's worldview, experiences, and feelings. They are also covert, meaning that they are not out in the open or readily available for others to see. Like the construction example, our boundaries tend to be buried within us and not openly accessible to others unless we reveal them. That said, the better we know someone, the more their behaviors and communication (verbal and nonverbal) will make covert boundaries more overt so that we can identify their boundaries and respect them. The same holds true for us: if we want people to respect our boundaries, we must make them more overt and communicate them openly.

In family therapy, specifically Structural Family therapy, boundaries are identified as "healthy" or "unhealthy" based on how well they are communicated and how members within the group can communicate and negotiate the rules of the boundaries (Goldenberg, Stanton, & Goldenberg, 2017). In other words, communicating about boundaries, making them more overt rather than covert, can help others to understand what you need. Boundaries are also defined by their permeability. Permeability in boundaries helps others understand how rigid or diffuse the boundary is and the degree to which the boundary might change. A rigid boundary tends to be fixed and unmovable; it is separate and distinct with little or no room to negotiate about the boundary. An example of this might be your bedtime. If you know that you are nonfunctional if you don't get a full eight hours of sleep, which means that you need to be in bed by 9:30 at night, then you will adhere to that boundary. If you are strict about that rule, not only by communicating it to others, but also by going to bed promptly at 9:30, then the boundary is considered rigid. When might a rigid boundary be considered unhealthy? When it is adhered to in the face of what could be considered an overriding issue, such as a sick member of the household who needs help, but you tell them, "So sorry, it's my bedtime. Good luck." I know you wouldn't do that.

The counterpoint to a rigid boundary is a diffuse one, which is characterized by blurred or indistinct rules and is easily violated because it isn't well defined. Using the same bedtime example, if you say that your bedtime is 9:30, but others can convince you to stay up later to watch a show or you are inconsistent in keeping that time frame (due to forces that you can control, not those you cannot, such as a sick household member), then the boundary is diffuse and easily changed or disrupted by both you and others. A way to think about a diffuse boundary gone awry is that if you don't respect and adhere to the boundary, then others won't either. When does a diffuse boundary become unhealthy? When you become angry or frustrated with others for not respecting a boundary that you don't respect or adhere to.

A healthy boundary has some flexibility; it can be negotiated and adapted as needed and allows for overriding issues and disruptions before becoming reestablished. Reflecting on your boundaries is important to the process that we are undertaking. The boundaries that you create so that you can live within your values and adhere to your flexible belief system can be the "make it or break it" part of living a life that is fully aligned and congruent with who you are at this phase of your life. Putting all this together, an example of how values, beliefs, and boundaries coalesce can be seen with nutrition. Maybe you're a person who puts a high value on good nutrition, which leads to a belief that healthy eating will lead to a healthy body. But if you become dogmatic in that belief and inflexible about what constitutes "good nutrition," you may find yourself engaging in very strict and rigid beliefs and boundaries around food. This rigidity could result in specific dieting rules that can be very limiting, such as never eating cupcakes or refined sugars, which may result in an unhealthy relationship with food.

The counterpoint—and healthier version of this alignment—is that you value good nutrition, you believe that healthy eating gives you a healthy body, and you maintain some *flexibility* in this belief, knowing that although you are eating healthy a great deal of the time, there are times when you will have less optimal choices or want to eat things that don't have the highest nutritional value, which is okay to do occasionally. This likely will lead to a more balanced relationship with food.

INTERNAL AND EXTERNAL FORCES

A great deal of wellness is about what you can control and is influenced by your values, beliefs, and boundaries. You are the hero of your midlife story, and part of being the hero means taking ownership of how you express these values through the dimensions of personal wellness. Reflection and change happen with small steps. In the rest of this book, we move through the following facets of wellness for you to reflect and consider how they impact your life: mental and emotional health, physical health (including fitness, nutrition, and sleep), appearance, intimate relationships, social health, vocation and career, leisure, and spiritual health and belief systems.

As we move forward, I'm asking you to be flexible. I'm asking you to reclaim your power and step outside of the boxes that you and others have created for you that likely no longer make sense at this stage of your life. I might ask you to do things that feel strange or silly, but by looking at each area of our lives, we can refine it so that we can redefine calm, purpose, and meaning in our lives.

CHAPTER THREE

MENTAL AND EMOTIONAL HEALTH

I returned to work two weeks after my dad died. Like most people who have suffered the death of a loved one, I was impaired. My grief reaction included memory issues, emotional outbursts, feelings of deep sadness and loss, crying spells, and a lack of energy and motivation. My first day back to work, I locked myself in my office and tried to respond to emails and get back up to speed on everything I had missed from the six weeks before his death. Those weeks were challenging, I worked from home and functioned as one of his caretakers. During the first two weeks after he died, I helped my mother plan as we both attempted to manage our grief and loss.

I got through my first morning crying spell at work and realized that it might be a good idea for me to call my doctor to see about getting a prescription for an antidepressant. I got lucky and was able to schedule a telehealth session during my lunch hour. I logged on to that session with my doctor and lost it, hysterically crying about the last few weeks, apologizing for crying, and promising that I had been doing everything that I could to cope with my loss in a healthy way. It was like I was trying to get an A in "good grieving." If I could say I was doing all the "right" things amid this loss, then I would somehow be rewarded for being super "healthy" during my grieving process. Anyway, she fully agreed that I would benefit from some medication, and after deciding which might be best, she let me know that the prescription would likely be ready for pickup later that day and I could take it as directed. What follows is the rest of the conversation:

Me: Oh, I'm not planning on taking that now. I'll take it in another four weeks once I've had a full six weeks to grieve.

My doctor: Um, what?

Me: I have my first therapy appointment in four weeks; it was the earliest I could get in. I am going to wait to take meds and really experience my grief naturally over the next four weeks.

My doctor: I appreciate that you have a lot of professional knowledge and practice in this area, but I think you might be using that to rationalize and control this situation in a way that might not be healthy for you.

Me: No, I'm good. I'll stick with the plan. I'll start taking meds in a few weeks and check back in. Thank you so much for talking me through this. [*Dissolves into more tears.*]

What are the lessons of this story? Obviously, I *was* trying to create control in an uncontrollable situation. I didn't have the mental space to accept that I was going through a major life crisis. I needed to stop and consider what I needed in that space and time. I also needed to realize (which I did shortly after this session) that it wasn't a controllable situation. Grief doesn't have an exact timeline, and when we experience a "once in a lifetime event" (my doctor's words), attempting to manage our emotions and our lives is an illusion that we create so that we can feel a semblance of control. One of the big questions that we grapple with in this chapter is how we can get help when our emotions are bigger than us. We'll also talk about smaller, less dramatic emotions and how we can respect what they are trying to tell us before they become bigger than we can manage.

In this chapter, we identify areas of dysregulation or misalignment in mental and emotional health, which often manifest in the form of stressors. First, we look at a way to conceptualize our stressors using the acronym "VUCA." Next, we examine the impact of external and internal stressors that influence mental health and review how values, beliefs, and boundaries can impact mental wellness. We also explore how issues in mental and emotional health can disguise themselves as issues in other areas. Finally, we consider the strategy of using an Eisenhower decision matrix to evaluate existing stressors to mental health and how this tool may help you to think about them differently.

Before going further, let's revisit the Global Assessment of Wellness (GAW) from chapter 2. There you were asked to rate on a 1–10 scale your satisfaction regarding your mental health, which encompasses your satisfaction with your overall emotional, psychological, and social well-being. Review your definition for the number you chose and what that score meant for you for this facet of wellness (both what you are and are not doing).

Now, consider the values sort that you completed in chapter 2. How do the ten values you selected align with mental and emotional health? Our mental and emotional health can impact what we value; what we value can impact our emotional and mental health. For example, if I value nonconformity and acceptance, then I may have some challenges regarding how I experience the world. Nonconformists often find themselves "outside" of the general population and sometimes feel less accepted than their more conforming peers. Feeling lonely or isolated when one wants to feel accepted can have a tremendous impact on mental health. Values can have reciprocal relationships with emotional health, and if our values don't fully align with each other, it can cause mental distress. Review the values you selected, examine how they impact your mental health, and determine whether they are aligned or misaligned in such a way that they create angst. There isn't necessarily an easy resolution if you identify a misalignment, but there is power in knowing that there might be and being able to identify when and how it occurs.

Finally, consider your beliefs about your values and the boundaries that you have created in life that help you to live out your values. Write only the values, beliefs, and boundaries that you believe pertain to mental and emotional health. Limit this list to only the top two or three; otherwise, it may begin to feel overwhelming. Use the values reflection exercise for your reflection; an example to guide you follows it.

VALUES REFLECTION EXERCISE

Values that encompass my mental and emotional wellness: _____

_____

_____

My beliefs about this value: _____
_____
_____
_____

The boundaries that help me live this value: _____
_____
_____
_____

SAMPLE VALUES REFLECTION

Values that encompass my mental and emotional wellness: *Kindness*

My beliefs about this value: *Kindness is something that everyone needs and deserves in their life; I try to be kind to those around me and hope that I am given kindness in return.*

The boundaries that help me live this value: *I will try to be kind to others even when they are not kind to me; showing kindness to others is about the person I want to be. I will give others the benefit of the doubt and show kindness until it is apparent that it is not received. I can be kind and not be a pushover.*

Now we need to consider what prevents you from living a fully well mental and emotional life. Aligning our values, beliefs, and boundaries helps us to create clarity about what we want. When we live outside of this alignment, it can create stress. For many of the women I work with, their stressors are what brings them to counseling and keeps them from living in alignment. Looking at table 3.1, what are the stressors in your life that keep you from living out your values in alignment with mental health and wellness? There may be a couple that come to mind but narrow your focus to just one or two for now and identify them below.

IDENTIFIED STRESSORS

Stressors that keep me from maintaining my mental/emotional health:

1. _____
2. _____

Keep these in mind as we move forward to discuss stressors and determine if they are external or internal.

CONCEPTUALIZING STRESSORS

Many stressors can be conceptualized by "VUCA," an acronym that describes four measures of understanding challenging situations. It stands for volatility, uncertainty, complexity, and ambiguity (Barber, 1992). *Volatility* refers to the probability of something being unpredictable and changeable, likely changing for the worse. In a stressful situation, we look for cues to see how changeable the situation is and if it will become worse. *Uncertainty*, or not knowing, could mean lacking enough information to attempt to predict an outcome. *Complexity* is the level of intricacy or difficulty that exists within the situation. And finally, *ambiguity* means that something can be understood in multiple ways or be subject to multiple interpretations. When experiencing stressors, we may subconsciously evaluate the experience using these metrics. Much like our discussion of boundary communication in chapter 2, making a stressor analysis overt and intentional may help us to evaluate our stressors in a new way so that we can create some perspective around them and gauge their impact on our lives.

Using VUCA to evaluate a stressor, let's consider the COVID-19 pandemic circa 2020, which was a highly volatile, highly uncertain, highly complex, and highly ambiguous situation. The constant change, which progressively worsened for a period of time, made it a volatile experience. This, coupled with the strain on medical and other resources, created a high-pressure, frightening situation. Uncertainty was an overriding emotion; the world had never encountered this virus before and didn't know how to handle it. The early days of the pandemic were complex and provided insight into how intricately woven and global a society we've become. Some may remember the global COVID transmission maps and travel restrictions. And finally, it was an ambiguous situation, understood in multiple ways, without any definitive or "right" answers about how to stop transmission in the early days, but rather several options that people had to choose from without the benefit of past experiences to guide them.

Contrast that example with COVID circa 2023, which was considered more of a low volatility, low uncertainty, moderately complex, low ambiguity situation. The COVID virus is now considered endemic and will be with us, like influenza and other viruses. Although the virus continues to mutate (like flu and other endemic diseases), the uncertainty surrounding it has decreased as scientists worldwide have been able to observe and study it over the last few years. COVID is still complex, even as volatility and uncertainty surrounding it have lessened. This complexity may be perceived as more manageable and less risky than it once was. Finally, although the course of this endemic disease varies among people, its treatment is better understood and managed because more is known about the virus and variant strains.

This illustration provides a good example for how to evaluate our stressors and a framework for understanding how a stressor can evolve. When we encounter a new or unique situation, we may experience a heightened response to it because we may interpret it as "high" by all VUCA measures. As we learn to understand and manage a stressor, its intensity may lessen because we understand it better and the situation becomes less uncertain and ambiguous. In midlife, we have the benefit of many more life experiences than we've ever had before. When we encounter something new, we may handle it better because we pull from our past experiences and competencies to manage the new problem. However, our past experiences don't always protect us from new experiences for which we are not prepared or chronic issues that require a lot of mental energy. Something else that is important to consider is whether the stressor is external or internal, as that may also help us to gauge how much control we have over a given situation.

EXTERNAL STRESSORS

External stressors have a great impact on our mental health and tend to be forces that are outside of us and beyond our control. My story at the beginning of this chapter describes an external stressor that caused great internal turmoil. What we can attempt to govern is our reaction, but as my example shows, attempts at control can range from irrational to healthier. Everyday external stress is one of the most common external forces that we deal with in our daily lives. Examples of everyday stress can include forgetting to put the trash out on garbage day (this morning) to a flight cancellation that causes a travel delay. Although these irritations can vary in their intensity, how we navigate everyday stress often depends on our overall resilience and resources. Individual resilience is the ability to adapt and recover from setbacks and is dependent upon the resources available to us to navigate setbacks. Resources can range from emotional support from others (such as an empathetic listener) to financial resources to help manage a problem (money for a hotel room while you're stranded in Dallas). Stress can have a cumulative effect on individuals, wherein the more incidents of stress you experience, the less resilient you are in the face of stress. A good metaphor for this is mosquito bites. One or two mosquito bites is a manageable irritation, but being swarmed with mosquitoes, getting twenty bites a day, every day for weeks on end can quickly become completely overwhelming.

Other external stressors that can impact and disrupt our mental and emotional health can include caregiver burden (children, elders), environmental changes impacting our quality of life, economic uncertainty, and community polarization and incivility regarding differing belief systems (e.g., political, religious, or healthcare views). With external stressors, we often must evaluate how to control our exposure to them and how to react to them in ways that align with our values and contribute positively to our mental health.

INTERNAL STRESSORS

Internal stressors originate within us; some of them are within our control and others are not. Internal manifestations of stress often center on our interpretation of our experiences, such as interpreting situations from a place of worry, anxiety, or existential dread.

That said, your internal experience of the world is typically predicated on two things: your nature and how you were nurtured. A descriptor for this is the saying "genetics loads the gun, and the environment pulls the trigger." This means that we all have genetic predispositions that may or may not express themselves, but our environments contribute a great deal to how our predispositions may manifest. Individuals who have more anxious traits don't necessarily manifest anxiety; however, if their environment feels unstable in some way, they may experience more anxiety than their peer who has a calmer temperament.

Some of our experience of internal stressors comes from our worldview and internalized beliefs that we have about the world. Note that in this context, "worldview" means your intellectual perspective about the world, and your internalized beliefs are the ways in which you integrate this information into how you think, feel, and act within the world. For example, if you have more often experienced the world as a safe place where you get the help you need when you need it, you may not be as likely to default to worry or anxiety when compared to a person who has not experienced a world that has given them the benefit of care and help. So, when thinking about your emotional and mental health in relation to internal stressors, you need to keep in mind your general temperament and how your worldview influences your experience of internal stressors.

Another thing to consider regarding internal stressors is how we can make them worse by worrying and overthinking them. Our brains are wired to keep us safe from danger, and both internal and external stressors pose dangers to us. With internal stressors, our brains recognize the stressor as a danger and activate our sympathetic nervous systems with "fight, flight, or freeze" responses. This is when our bodies begin to have a stress reaction, such as tense muscles and higher heart and respiratory rates, among other responses. Our brains are programmed, through evolution, to keep us alive in natural environments. However, many issues that we deal with in our modern world are not "natural world" dangers; they are more abstract but just as important to our survival. They are not the immediate danger of a tiger standing in our path;

they are typically the existential danger of our lives changing or being out of control in some way. Our very smart brain can't tell the difference between a real tiger and what I call a "ghost tiger," which isn't an animal in front of us, but rather a trigger in our brains that elicits the same reaction that a real tiger would. Many of the internal stressors that we deal with are "ghost tigers," which our brain interprets as just as powerful as real tigers and that trigger the same physical and emotional response that physical dangers can.

Ghost tigers manifest in our heads through our worry, existential dread, anxiety, and depression and trigger an automatic stress reaction (Kabat-Zinn, 2013). We've all experienced this when we are up at 3:00 a.m., staring at the ceiling and thinking or worrying about some issue that feels very important. We experience all of the physical manifestations of a real threat, such as racing thoughts, increased heart rate, shallow breathing, and so on. Our brains are preparing us for a fight when we're lying in bed and it is time to rest. When we get stuck in a state of worry, we are feeding the tiger. Telling ourselves to relax is a nice idea but typically isn't helpful when we're in this state. In a bit, we explore the types of help that are available when we're overwhelmed due to our internal stressors.

A COLLISION OF EXTERNAL AND INTERNAL STRESSORS

Eleanor came to therapy due to her experience of external and internal stressors, which centered on the decision to have children. She was in her late thirties and was struggling with her and her partner's discussions about having a biological child. She had a great deal of fear and uncertainty about global warming and environmental changes that could threaten the stability of the world. Eleanor described her struggles with watching the news and reading scientific reports about how the earth could become increasingly inhospitable to life during the coming decades. She also disclosed that she struggles with depression and existential angst for herself; these personal issues in addition to the responsibility for another human in the face of an environmental crisis felt like more than she could manage. She said at one point, "I already have my own issues; I'm not sure if I can bring a child into this world with that and all of these other crises happening on top of it." What brought her to counseling was her experiences of her internal stressors of depression and anxiety and her external stressors via news reports, which triggered additional emotional and physical responses.

When we looked at the values she was struggling with, one of them was family and another was stability. Although Eleanor loved the idea of family, it also created a lot of uncertainty and ambiguity for her; she didn't know how she could function as a mother and partner with her preexisting issues. She valued stability, which means that she put a great deal of effort into creating a life with low volatility, uncertainty, and ambiguity. She acknowledged that her life was complex and that was okay because she had learned to manage the complexity over time. Eleanor's belief about having a family was that she couldn't have children and the type of stability that she craved. The external stressor of environmental issues contributed to her existential angst and amplified her fear of the unknown. The boundary that she created to manage her anxiety and fear around family and stability was to avoid conversations about children with her partner, but it was slowly building into resentment between the two of them.

What she realized in her counseling sessions is that her internal existential angst and fear of external stressors (e.g., environmental change) combined to create a situation in which she was avoiding her life rather than living it. Eleanor was frozen in a state of ambivalence that left her stuck. She had some questions to grapple with. What were her overriding motivations? How was her fear stopping her from doing what she wanted to do? What could she control? She could accept that her anxiety was getting the best of her and that she needed to tap into some additional coping skills and resources to manage it differently. Eleanor also wanted to explore her desire and motivation for having children, putting aside the things that were holding her back so that she could embrace what excited her about having children: "I want to coparent with my partner." Eleanor's turning point happened when she realized that the way she was handling both her external and internal stressors was stopping her from living her life. She chose to continue to process her issues so that she could live her authentic life. She was brave to ask for help and try new skills to manage her internal stressors so that she could work through her beliefs around her external values and stressors and ultimately attempt to move forward in her life.

BE BRAVE: ASK FOR HELP

Just like Eleanor, we all have areas in our lives where we need to ask for help. Sometimes we try to control the narrative when we ask for help, like I did while I was grieving. Or we learn to trust and let go of our need to control when we realize that asking for help can give us some of the mental relief and release that we need. When you're gauging how much help you need, it's important to remember *which stressors are reasonably within your control.* Those may be things for which you need to make different choices, and in so doing, they will cease to be issues in your life. Other stressors take more work to negotiate and may never go away fully; however, finding the right supports to help manage those stressors can go a long way in making life a bit easier.

Finding the right support can come down to asking for help; I say that knowing that asking for help can be one of the hardest and most vulnerable acts for many people. The act of asking can go different ways: we might not get what we want, but we get something that helps; we get what we need; or we get little or no help and feel even more despondent about our issues. Becoming more upset and experiencing our frustration for a short amount of time is okay; getting stuck in them and allowing it to keep us from moving forward is a problem.

When we're asking for help, we must think about who or what the best supports might be in each situation. Asking for help for something that is within your control may not be the best use of a resource. One example might be asking someone else to remind you to drink more water for your health. First, you've given responsibility for your behavior to someone else, who can't control your behavior. Second, you've asked someone to help you do something that you might be able to do in another way, such as setting reminders on your phone or using an accountability app. Resources such as people and relationships are not infinite, so it is important to be mindful of what we're asking for. For things that are reasonably within our control, we need to think about how we can be personally accountable rather than drawing on our human resources in those situations.

It's realistic to ask for help when something isn't working in your life to the point that it causes distress. I frame this for clients in terms of bravery: "something wasn't working in your life, and it was so uncomfortable you came to a stranger, albeit a professional, for help. That is a powerful indicator of how much it is bothering you." Asking for help typically means that we have moved beyond our problem-solving skills and are experiencing a level of distress that makes it necessary to look outside of ourselves for a possible solution. Depending on the level of distress, we may seek different types of support.

For many of us, talking to our friends and people we trust is a great way to process what is troubling us and find meaning or possible solutions to problems. However, when our problems become bigger and less manageable, we may seek help from some other source because we want to explore our issues privately. Ways to explore our problems can include community support such as spiritual or religious organizations, professional helpers, medical professionals, reading books or listening to podcasts about certain issues, or considering medication intervention. Sometimes it can feel very challenging to determine how critical a stressor is; what follows is a tool that may help as you're trying to figure out how stressors may be impacting you.

A ROADMAP TO DECISION MAKING

The Eisenhower matrix was created by Dwight D. Eisenhower to prioritize tasks. It is often used in business and management to organize tasks in terms of importance. In this case, it can be used to examine our stressors and how important they are in our lives. Table 3.1 shows a decision matrix.

Table 3.1. Sample Decision Matrix

	Urgent	Not Urgent
Important	Do (*stressors with deadlines or consequences*):	Schedule (*stressors with unclear deadlines but that are important to long-term success or happiness*):
Not Important	Delegate (*stressors that need to be addressed but for which you may not have the specific skill set*):	Delete (*stressors that are distractions or unnecessary*):

Using my life as an example, here are four stressors that align with the quadrants of the matrix.

1. Maintaining the yard
2. Keeping up with friends and family through social media
3. Working through my emotional grief after my father's death
4. Attending to the funny noise the HVAC system was making last summer

In table 3.2 you can see how I prioritized each task and determined its importance.

Table 3.2. Sample Decision Matrix

	Urgent	Not Urgent
Important	Do: Take medication and attend counseling sessions to process my grief. Otherwise, I'm not functional. (*Employs both external help and internal responsibility*)	Schedule: Make an appointment with the HVAC company; I live in the South and summer without AC is not good. (*Employs external help*)
Not Important	Delegate: Ask my husband to take care of the yard; this may mean that he does it or delegates it to a lawn service. (*Employs external help*)	Delete: Maintaining social media accounts. This is a personal decision for everyone, but social media is not healthy for me. (*Employs internal responsibility*)

Yes, I conveniently gave you stressors that fit into the boxes, and no, life rarely fits into easy boxes. However, I have seen this exercise work for people because it forces them to evaluate stressors and prioritize how they manage them. We don't have a lot of time on the planet, and we certainly don't want to spend our precious time negotiating stressful things. That said, a couple of comments about my matrix above: Notice that I indicate whether an item requires external help or is an internal responsibility. The items that were highly dependent upon my behavior and my compliance with boundaries I set for myself are internal responsibilities; those for which I need external help are marked as such because they involve another person or entity that I am dependent on to execute the task.

For example, taking medication and maintaining therapy appointments is my responsibility and I can't do it without the professionals who are helping, therefore it requires both external help and internal responsibility. Something that I appreciate about this matrix is that it includes a "delete" section. I value being close with my family and friends but using social media as the mechanism to maintain those relationships didn't align with my beliefs that visits, calls, and video chats are a more satisfying way to connect with others. Also, I found it challenging to maintain time boundaries using social media. For me, it is a time suck, and I would lose hours of my life looking at things that were not remotely related to my loved ones, therefore I chose to "delete" this for now.

DECISION MATRIX EXERCISE

Remember those two stressors from the beginning of the chapter, the ones that prevent you from living your most healthy emotional life? How might they fit into this decision matrix? Using table 3.3, complete your decision matrix using your defined stressors.

Table 3.3. Decision Matrix Exercise

	Urgent	Not Urgent
Important	Do: _____ _____ _____ _____ _____	Schedule: _____ _____ _____ _____ _____
Not Important	Delegate: _____ _____ _____ _____ _____	Delete: _____ _____ _____ _____ _____

As you evaluate where your stressors fit, also ask yourself if they require external help, internal responsibility, or both. If you need external help, consider what kind of external help you need. This may include individuals who are close to you, such as a friend, partner, or family member. It may also include individuals or entities that are not as close to you, such as professional service workers, colleagues, helpers, or clergy members. Also consider that getting help sometimes means that you're not seeking out people, but ideas. This can include internet searches, books, podcasts, or other resources to help you. Finally, sometimes additional help includes medical interventions such as medication, outpatient care, dietetics appointments, and so forth.

Internal responsibilities can be more challenging because they rely on our self-discipline and willpower, which is finite. Sometimes we need help maintaining internal responsibilities through using automated reminders (like for drinking more water), accountability partners (like a workout partner you meet for your walk), or by giving yourself grace and self-forgiveness when you're not able to maintain them for some reason. Something helpful that I do when trying to self-motivate to maintain an internal responsibility is to repeat the mantra, "A promise to the self is sacred." One of my teachers taught me this mantra and I find it to be a powerful tool when I'm avoiding something and attempting to pull my self-discipline together so I can move forward. As we end this chapter, consider the reflection questions below.

REFLECTION QUESTIONS

- What's one thing you know you need help with?
- What can you control yourself?
- What do you need to ask for help with?
- Whom do you need to ask for help from?
- Write out what you want to ask for.

CHAPTER FOUR

PHYSICAL HEALTH

EARLY DETECTION SAVES LIVES

I'm a rule follower, and if you tell me I'm supposed to do something that benefits my health, I follow through. Which is how I found myself having my first mammogram very shortly after my fortieth birthday. For those ladies who haven't had their mammogram yet and are late to the party, welcome! However, the story that follows may not inspire too many appointments.

So there I am, boob in the big machine, my gown hanging open in front of the polite stranger who is making small talk with me. I've had people describe having a mammogram as feeling like your breast is being slammed between two cold refrigerator doors. My experience is more like when you pinch your finger between two binder prongs and you're trying to pull the skin out toward freedom. Not horribly painful, but not what I'd choose to do on my afternoon off. I digress....

As I held my breath so the tech could take images, she told me that after my pictures were reviewed by the doctor, I would receive a letter in the mail letting me know that I had a normal mammogram and a reminder to make an appointment next year. The next thought through my head was, *Wow, I really wish I was going to get one of those letters, but I'm not.* There was no reason for me to think this. I have very few risk factors and a limited family history of breast cancer. Yet that thought was thrown into the universe.

Fast forward to the next day during a meeting when I received a call from the breast center letting me know that I would have to make an appointment to come back because they detected some tissue that was hard to read. What was my availability in the next few days? I remember looking at my boss as I was taking the call and seeing the sympathy fill her eyes. If something like this has ever happened to you, you understand the horrifying anxiety spiral that occurred for me next. If not, then I hope it never happens to you.

What followed from my baseline mammogram was about two years of follow-ups, mammograms, sonograms, a biopsy, a benign lumpectomy, appointments with a breast surgeon, and interactions with insurance companies about my preexisting conditions, risk factors, and eligibility for certain preventative care, such as breast MRIs. Do I feel good about following the mammogram "rule" and engaging in preventative care at an early age? Yes. But the outcomes forever changed how I think of health and what it means to be physically well.

What I experienced in my first mammogram and the treatments that followed challenged my belief that as a person who strives to be healthy, maintain good habits, and take care of myself, I will be automatically rewarded with a clean bill of health for as long as I'm alive. People in my family don't get sick often, and even when they are, they deny it and suffer in silence. This familial denial creates an unrealistic expectation that I'll always be healthy, and when I ran into a situation where I wasn't fully "healthy," it caused a lot of distress. I had done everything (mostly) right. I tried to eat healthy, exercise, meditate, maintain healthy relationships, all the things. The harsh truth is that even when we try to do everything we can to prevent illnesses, we can't control all of the external and internal forces at work in our bodies that influence our health. Does this mean that we stop doing the things that keep us feeling good and maintain our health? No. But it does help us put into perspective our "why" for maintaining our physical health and the benefits and limits that a healthy lifestyle can have on our overall life experience.

Our goals in this chapter are to identify where you're experiencing dysregulation and misalignment in your physical health. We broaden the definition to include fitness, nutrition, sleep, and medical care. We also look at typical health changes that take place in midlife and the role that stress plays in our physical health. Like the last chapter, we examine how we're impacted by both internal and external factors that can influence this domain of health. Before we go further, let's review your satisfaction with your physical health from the global assessment of wellness exercise in chapter 2.

GLOBAL ASSESSMENT OF PHYSICAL WELLNESS EXERCISE

Physical health: Satisfaction includes your ability to recover from illness and the state of your physical body and its operations (base your score on things that you can control as well as those you cannot)

1   5   10

Review your definition for the number you chose and what that score meant for you on this facet of wellness (both what you are and are not doing) and summarize it below.

Physical health score

    Definition of score: _____

    What this score means to me: _____

To expand upon this exercise, explore the values, beliefs, and boundaries that you have created in your life that impact your physical health. Write these out for yourself in the physical health values, beliefs, and boundaries exercise that follows; your answers can help guide you through the rest of the chapter.

PHYSICAL HEALTH VALUES, BELIEFS, AND BOUNDARIES EXERCISE

Values that encompass my physical wellness: _____

_____

_____

My beliefs about these values: _____

_____

_____

The boundaries that help me live these values: _____

_____

_____

Many midlife women with whom I work value physical health, but their ability to tend to it varies. Reasons for avoiding or ignoring health include lacking time, issues related to perfectionism, costs/money, no or limited health insurance, lack of options for activities or care, and forces outside of their control (such as caregiving responsibilities). All these legitimate concerns can factor into our ability to influence our physical health, in particular lack of resources, such as being able to secure and afford medical care, has a significant influence over one's ability to maintain wellness. I wish that I had an answer or a magic wand that could change this circumstance for others. Having worked in a hospital setting, I know how devastating it can be to balance the need for medical care against the costs. In this book, I focus on low- or no-cost activities that are easily done at home or in your community. But first, let's talk about typical changes that occur in midlife.

THE ONLY CONSTANT IS CHANGE

Here's the thing about our physical bodies as we enter midlife: we are just getting used to them! In our earlier years, if we're fortunate, we can well predict what our bodies will do and how they function. Most of us understand and know our physical exertion abilities, are physically active in the ways that we want, and understand our physical limitations. We understand our hormonal and menstrual cycles (as well as they can be understood), we know what our bodies are capable of in terms of sex and having children, our senses are in good working order, and we've grown into our body's shape and understand what it takes to maintain it.

And then, at some point in the middle years, things begin to change. Physically our bodies don't build muscle the way that they used to, and we may find that our metabolism has slowed, which can lead to unexpected weight changes. We may also find that our ability to maintain certain physical activities has changed due to wear and tear on our bodies or decreasing stamina. We may also find that some of our senses are different, such as changes in eyesight or hearing. And finally, we may begin to experience signs and symptoms of perimenopause and menopause.

I am not telling you anything that you don't know, but isn't it funny how we can fool ourselves into believing that the natural progression of aging is going to happen to everyone but us? And then when it does start to happen, we're outraged. *Okay, I was outraged.* It began when I was diagnosed with arthritis in one of my feet, which eventually changed the way that I exercised and the types of shoes that I wore. It took a long time for me to accept that this was just the beginning of a long series of experiences that would occur over my lifespan and that my body is going to change and will degrade as I continue to get older. Let me not be overly dramatic—my foot isn't falling off—but I know that if I want to live an active physical life, I have to cut out high-impact exercises and super-high heels.

The changes we experience in our physical health in our middle years can feel unpredictable, like what we went through when we transitioned from childhood into adolescence. In this case, it could be that we're experiencing changes in certain abilities that may lead us to feel sad, frightened, or angry. For some, going through menopause feels like the loss of their worth as women. Some changes might make us happy. For example, ultimately I was not sad to leave high-impact cardio behind. The takeaway is that there will be change; accepting it and adapting is important so that we can continue to live well. These are the internal aspects of physical health. We're also impacted by external factors, a major one being stress, which we discussed in chapter 1. Although many factors can contribute to stress in our lives, it's important that we also understand the impact that it has on our physical bodies, the consequences of which can create greater health issues than we may realize.

THE PRICE THE BODY PAYS

Allostatic load is a term that was coined in 1993 by researchers McEwen and Stellar to describe the relationship between stress and factors that lead to disease. When our bodies are confronted with stressors, they can react through multiple systems: behaviorally, neurochemically (interaction between the nervous and endocrine systems), through our endocrine system (certain glands may overproduce hormones to maintain body system stability), neurologically (damage to neurons in our brains), and through our immune system (which is designed to fight off diseases). When the body is confronted with stressors, it works very hard to maintain stability. The body adapts by fluctuating physiological responses in the systems listed above to meet the external demand the body encounters; this fluctuation is called *allostasis* (McEwen & Stellar, 1993). A real-world example of bodily adaptation to maintain stability is seen in cortisol secretion, which is a hormone that is released when individuals experience stress. Cortisol released into the body is a normal body reaction; it is the "fight or flight" hormone that prepares us to survive in challenging situations. Remember the "ghost tiger" conversation in the last chapter? Here she is again. When we experience long-term exposure to stress, one of the side effects can be an overproduction of cortisol. Cortisol has a number of effects on the body, including regulating your blood sugar levels, blood pressure, inflammatory responses, and controlling your sleep-wake cycle.

This important hormone is intended for short-term use only; cortisol helps us survive life-threatening situations. Think about a stress response: heightened blood pressure, alertness (to the point of not being able to rest or sleep), surges in energy, and lessening of feelings of pain or bodily discomfort. However, if the stressors are sustained for long periods of time, then the body continues to release cortisol in an attempt to sustain the fight or flight response. Long-term effects of cortisol are not as beneficial as the short-term effects. In the long term, excessive cortisol can lead to higher blood pressure, inflammation, disruption in sleep cycles, and weight gain (Moyer et al., 1994).

Allostatic load can be understood as the price the body pays to maintain stability in the face of stressors. In their work, McEwen and Stellar state that there are genetic and environmental factors that influence how individuals react to stressors. Some of these factors are within our control and some are not. What the researchers suggest is that individuals minimize exposure to stress and engage in activities that can help combat the physical health consequences that can arise in the face of stress. One fascinating aspect of this initial work is that it led to additional research, which shows that there is a relationship between genetics and environmental factors that can lead to differences in how individuals develop (or don't develop) diseases. What makes these findings important is that we can attempt to control certain behaviors, which, in turn, can help alleviate some of the negative consequences of stress and possibly how we experience diseases.

Here's why I love the concept of allostatic load: it gives a name to what we inherently know. Prolonged stress is not good; it can have negative consequences for our physical health. It is not a badge of honor that demonstrates how important or worthwhile we are. Although we can't control all the factors that contribute to disease, understanding allostatic load and health factors that we can control gives us a way to make informed decisions so we can live our healthiest life. The thing that we can control is our behavior, which directly relates to our values, beliefs, and boundaries. Allostatic load also gives us a way to think about how our physical health experiences can be negatively compounded or made worse when we don't take care of ourselves. For example, if you are a person who has a high-stress life, you may find that you engage in high-risk behaviors, such as excessive drinking and eating unhealthy foods to cope. These behaviors increase the likelihood of physical consequences, such as high blood pressure and cholesterol. People with high blood pressure and cholesterol are at higher risk for heart disease and stroke. In this example, your body is working hard to maintain stability in the face of these issues and has a higher allostatic load. Compare this to a person who has a high-stress life and attempts to minimize high-risk behaviors, walks to manage stress, and attempts to eat balanced food choices. They also may have high blood pressure and cholesterol, and they are proactively engaging in behaviors that can help their body better maintain stability and may therefore have a lower allostatic load.

As stewards of our physical health, the behaviors that we can work to control include our mindset, sleep, eating, and movement. In the next section, I offer some suggestions for life tweaks in each of these areas that can help you refine how you care for your body. These are proactive changes you can make in small steps, which can have a big impact on how you feel. Consider the physical health value that you wrote at the beginning of this chapter; it may be that one of these tweaks can help you to expand how you live within your beliefs and boundaries of this value.

WHAT WE CAN DO

Mindset

I began this chapter with a tale of preventative care that ultimately benefited me, even though the journey was scary. As a woman, it sometimes feels as though I have more things in my body that can "go wrong" than my male counterparts. Maybe this is why I hear from so many women that they sometimes avoid attending to medical care even though they know it is important. I originally titled this section "preventative care" because one of the things that we can control is going to our doctors. But the more I thought about what influences how we care for our physical health, the more I realized how important mindset is. Specifically, how we manage shame, ambiguity, and our inner critic.

I work with a lot of women who know they need to work out, to go to the doctor, or to eat differently, but something stops them. The thing that they don't say is the word *shame*. Shame, as defined by Brené Brown (2021), "is the intensely painful feeling or experience of believing that we are flawed and therefore unworthy of love, belonging, and connection." I believe that there are too many women who feel shame when they think about their bodies. For example, many women fear going to medical appointments because they already feel some internalized shame about their bodies; going to a medical expert to be examined and possibly told about health issues that we "should" be able to fix can feed into this sense of shame.

Ambiguity made its appearance in chapter 3 when we discussed VUCA (volatility, uncertainty, complexity, and ambiguity), and here it is again. In this case, ambiguity has to do with the fact that sometimes when it comes to our bodies, there are no "right" answers. I was speaking with a friend the other day who is having some health issues for which her doctors can't give her a definitive diagnosis. She is becoming increasingly frustrated because she doesn't feel well, and she isn't able to receive guidance about how she can improve her situation. I think there is a commonly held belief that medical professionals can give us answers and a plan to improve every ailment that we can suffer from. Although we are certainly better off with current medical knowledge than we were a hundred years ago, many physical issues can occur in our bodies that our medical professionals don't have an answer for, which is both scary and frustrating.

In the face of ambiguity is the realization that although we don't have the answers we crave, we still must keep living our lives to the best of our ability. When it comes to our physical health, this can mean concentrating once again on the things that we can control and that our inner wisdom tells us is right. In the case of my friend, her answer was to concentrate on lowering the number of inflammatory foods and chemicals that she was exposing her body to. Will this help her? It probably won't hurt her; it might be one of the issues contributing to how she's feeling (no one can say for sure); and it gives her something that she can work toward that gives her a sense of control, which is ultimately what we want in a situation that feels chaotic.

It has been said that perfectionism drives our *inner critic*. Perfectionism can be seen as a defense mechanism that protects us from our perception of others' judgment by making our actions above reproach. Every defense mechanism has positive and negative aspects. The positive side of perfectionism includes "perfectionistic striving," which is characterized by attempting to achieve high standards. The negative side is "perfectionistic concern," which includes engaging in self-criticism (the inner critic), fear of failure, and perceived or real negative evaluation by self or others (Stoeber & Otto, 2006).

You don't have to identify as a perfectionist to have an inner critic, but in my experience people who have high anxiety and tend to be perfectionistic struggle more with this issue. Here's where it all goes awry: when your inner critic starts to create emotional distress due to unreasonable self-expectations and you're unable to accept your present circumstances and limitations. For example, a client of mine was an avid rock climber. However, due to health issues, she was unable to train or engage in climbing for an extended period. When she did go back to the gym, she found that she was not physically able to climb like she wanted to due to muscle loss, weight gain, and being out of practice. My client had a picture in her head of where she had been before she stopped climbing and was very frustrated by her lack of progress at the gym because she was not where she believed she "should" be. Her biggest struggle wasn't starting up her training routine or practicing climbing. Her biggest struggle was her inner critic.

According to their 2015 study, James, Verplanken, and Rimes found that unhealthy perfectionism that results in distress is influenced by higher levels of self-criticism. The more you have perfectionistic tendencies and the more you listen to your inner critic, the more likely you are to experience higher levels of emotional distress. It tends to be that people experiencing emotional distress attempt to find ways to stop the discomfort. I have seen individuals handle this by either quitting what they're doing because it seems to be the only way to silence the inner critic or striving to the point of exhaustion to reach an unattainable goal.

In the case of my client, she found that she was avoiding going to the gym so that she didn't have to listen to her inner critic. We did some work on countering her negative self-talk with compassion, observing the present moment without emotional attachment, and examining her self-judgments with realistic observation. One of the outcomes of this work was to quiet her inner critic and to listen to what it might be trying to tell her. In this case, what she uncovered is that although she enjoyed movement and exercise, she no longer enjoyed climbing the way she had before her break. We discussed the difference between quitting because of her inner critic and stopping climbing because she wanted to; this was an important distinction because quitting and stopping were two different things for her: quitting meant that she was frustrated and couldn't succeed at climbing, whereas stopping meant that she knew she could climb if she continued to try but she wanted to step away because the activity wasn't serving her the way it once did.

Combating shame, ambiguity, and the inner critic takes time, work, and consistency. It can start with noticing and recording when you are engaging in negative self-talk. This can be as simple as starting a list on your phone and noting when you engage in negative self-talk; doing this for a week can be a powerful way to see how often you engage in this behavior and what the negativity is about. Second, engaging in greater self-compassion can help. This means that when a negative thought comes up—"I didn't do enough today"—you counter it with self-compassion—"I did the things that I had energy for today, the rest will wait until tomorrow." Additional self-compassion exercises can include using loving kindness meditation practices, which guide you through a practice of self-acceptance and care.

Managing emotional distress when you are experiencing ambiguity about your physical health can be very challenging, but one tool that I've used with clients is to create a "worry time" in their day. Worry time can be about five minutes every day when you put on a timer and worry about all the things that you need to. When the timer goes off, worry time is over. If you think about the worry outside of the official worry time, you tell yourself, "It's not worry time; I can't think about this right now." This technique is something called *thought blocking*, in which we attempt to disrupt intrusive thoughts.

We also can listen to what the inner critic is trying to tell us about how we feel. This mechanism is often the voice that is trying to push us away from feelings of vulnerability or shame. When we take the time to be curious about what we're feeling and examine it in a nonjudgmental way, it can help us to have a greater sense of what is troubling us. Getting in touch with our inner vulnerability and shame and accepting it as part of who we are is imperative to be fully aligned and congruent with how we think, feel, and behave. Finally, we also must accept that we may never fully silence the inner critic; rather, our work is to soften the voice of the critic and allow it to become a messenger of our feelings rather than the driver of our identity.

Sleep

Sleep is as imperative to our health and survival as food, water, and air. However, sometimes we treat lack of sleep as a badge of honor: "I got by with just four hours of sleep yesterday." Or we are so busy trying to get everything in our lives done that we forgo sleep to complete tasks: "I don't have time to sleep, that's why I stay up until 2:00 am to get everything done." Regardless of the reason, sleep disturbances are serious because they can impact our overall physical and mental health.

It's a common belief that in midlife women suffer from sleep disturbances and a decline in the amount of sleep that they can enjoy. For example, a 2021 report published in the journal *Menopause* found that new onset sleep problems that occur in midlife were associated with risks of increased unemployment and approximately $2 billion per year in lost productivity in the United States (Kagan, Shiozawa, Epstein, & Espinosa, 2021). In contrast, we can also look to research completed in 2020 in the journal *Sleep*, which found that a small sample of women (three hundred) did not experience the sleep disturbances that are attributed to women during their middle years (Matthews et al., 2020). Two studies on midlife women's sleep, and two very different findings.

What does this mean for you? Honestly, it means that there is no definitive answer that fits everyone. You may fall into one of these two camps: you have sleep issues that are creating problems in your life, or you're not experiencing sleep issues, and everything is fine. What I have found as a counselor is that since the pandemic, more individuals are experiencing at least some mild issues of sleep disturbance, including trouble getting to and staying asleep, and occasional insomnia. That said, lack of sleep is a medical issue that should be treated by a professional, so please seek help if you have more serious issues that are impairing your ability to engage in activities of daily living.

For many folks I work with, evaluating their overall sleep hygiene and making modifications to their sleep habits can do wonders for their ability to get good rest. *Sleep hygiene* is a term that is used to describe both the behaviors and the environment where you sleep. Goals of good hygiene include maintaining a sleep routine, setting bedtimes and waking times, creating and following a bedtime routine, maintaining healthy habits that promote sleep, and making sure that your sleeping environment is optimal.

Let's start with setting bedtimes and wake times. We all enjoy "sleeping in" when we don't have any duties in the morning. Be it a weekend or holiday, sleeping in is as close to feeling like a kid who just got out for summer break as I get these days. Although changing your sleep times occasionally is okay, drastically changing or altering your sleep schedule between workdays and non-workdays is difficult. It's hard to get back into a "routine" from one to the other because you're constantly seesawing back and forth, which can leave you feeling tired, fatigued, sluggish from too much or little sleep, and not as present as you would like to be.

The second goal is setting a bedtime routine like you had when you were a kid. That routine served the purpose of creating a set of habits that mentally and physically prepared you for going to sleep. Your routine can include putting on your pajamas, washing your face, dimming the lights, or drinking calming tea. Part of your habit also can be incorporating some time to decompress from your day, which might include playing some soft music, meditating, praying, reading, or other types of activities that help you relax before bedtime.

Creating an optimal environment for sleep includes creating a space that is devoted to rest and sleep. If your sleeping space doubles as a work or hobby space, it can create distraction when you're trying to rest. Some ways to help with this are to have a place where you can put away or hide your work items so that they are not visually distracting you. I had a client who created a ritual after her work hours of putting away her laptop in a drawer at the end of the day so she could create a boundary between her work time and home time, and it turned out to be a simple and effective habit. Perhaps also consider creating a technology/media-free zone during your pre-bedtime routine so that your brain can disconnect from these types of stimuli.

How does your daytime routine impact your ability to sleep? Important daylight activities that we don't think about but that can impact our sleep quality include:

- getting enough daylight/sunlight exposure, which helps maintain our circadian rhythms
- being physically active during the day
- reducing and limiting nicotine and alcohol intake
- reducing and limiting caffeine intake in the afternoon and evening
- eating at a time that allows your body to digest before you want to go to bed

Finally, make sure that you use your bed for sleep and intimacy. It's important that your brain associates your bed with sleep so that it is easier to reinforce your routine. Using any of these sleep hygiene habits can help you to get more rest. Attempting to build them into your habits over time (e.g., by incorporating one new habit a month over six months) may just revolutionize how you rest.

Food

We must eat; it is part of our survival. However, as we enter midlife our relationship with food and diet can become challenging. Physiologically, during midlife, our bodies are changing due to perimenopause and menopause, which can impact our bodies due to a drop in estrogen production. The results of this hormonal drop can be related to a larger amount of body fat accumulation (particularly in the midsection), reduced metabolism, increased body inflammation, blood pressure, and cholesterol, and decreased bone density and muscle mass. As one study stated, "Menopause signifies a critical intervention point for risk screening and individual lifestyle modifications for managing these issues and ensuring healthy longevity" (Feskens et al., 2022, p. 10). One of the lifestyle modifications that can be important during midlife is how and what we are eating, otherwise known as our nutritional intake. Key components to consider when thinking about nutrition at this stage are foods that can cause inflammation, the types and amounts of food in our diet, and our relationship with food.

Inflammation

Our diet is important throughout our lifespan, but in midlife, it has the potential to set the stage for how healthily we age. What we eat can impact our internal systems; for example, if we eat a lot of foods that can cause inflammation, such as sugar, red meat, or processed carbohydrates, we may find that we are susceptible to related health issues such as increased risk for heart disease, type 2 diabetes, or stroke. Increased intake of inflammatory foods has also been linked to impairments in learning and memory for individuals across the lifespan (Stevenson, 2017). There are long-term risks and benefits to our nutritional choices that can affect us later in life; the good news is that it is one of the behaviors that we can augment and change in small ways that can make a big impact.

Signs of inflammation in the body can include one or more symptoms, which can include general pain or specific pain like joint pain, abdominal pain, or chest pain, fatigue and tiredness, and rashes. These symptoms can either be precursors to chronic diseases or co-occur with certain illnesses. According to research, foods that can have anti-inflammatory properties include fish, dark leafy greens, fruits, vegetables, olive oil, and certain spices like turmeric. Foods like these may help you to feel better; however, radical changes in diet can be a shock to your system. You may want to consider more research on beneficial foods and integrating changes slowly, like swapping regular vegetable oil for olive oil when cooking.

Types and Amounts of Food

Many of us remember learning about the food pyramid in school; the revised version is called "MyPlate," which the US Department of Agriculture (USDA) introduced in 2011. The USDA's revised guidelines provide information on healthy eating across the lifespan but generally recommends that approximately half of one's plate have fruits and vegetables, a quarter of a plate have grains (at least half of which contain whole grains), a quarter have some type of protein (plant or animal based), with a small side plate of low-fat or fat-free dairy. What I like about the visual of the plate is that it gives us a real-life way to envision the types of foods to eat and the proportions in which to eat them.

We've already discussed how certain foods may create inflammation in the body; these also tend to be foods that are higher in calories and lower in overall nutritional benefit. I love a good candy bar, and when I eat one, I need to be aware that the sugar and calories I'm consuming may be feeding my body and giving me short-term energy but will leave me hungry and cranky after I crash from the sugar rush. Less refined foods (like the ones found around the perimeter of the grocery store) tend to be the ones that are the healthiest but that also require some additional creativity and time for preparation.

While writing this chapter, I consulted with my friend and colleague, Amy, about dietetics. Amy is a registered dietician who works in a medical setting and offers education sessions for medical and mental health providers regarding the impact of food and diet. She reminded me of an old habit we used to have during our monthly brunches. We went to a restaurant that offered a carafe of mimosas, which made for a great visit. We would sit, drink, and eat for at least an hour and a half, catching up on our lives. Inevitably, we would go home from these brunches feeling tired and cranky—we often would text later that day about how tired we felt. What we didn't realize, until a carafe was prepared in front of us at one brunch, was that we were sharing an entire bottle of prosecco every time we met!

We were not used to consuming that much alcohol, which illustrates the power of "hidden" ingredients and calories. This is especially true with alcoholic beverages, wherein a serving size for wine is five and a half ounces, not the nine ounces we typically get in restaurants. These additional calories add up over time and significantly impact your health. Other places where we can find hidden ingredients include excessive sugars in certain foods (such as tomato-based products) or additional fats in items that are considered lower in sugar (such as yogurts).

Because healthy nutrition habits set us up for positive long-term health, making gradual changes like reducing the amounts of sugars and fats we consume and reevaluating our food portion sizes can be important as we age. If we know that our metabolism slows as we age, we may want to think about how much we eat. Food is energy, and if you consume more energy than you're burning, your body stores the excess energy in the form of fat. If you are active and engage in a good deal of movement, you'll want to adjust your food (energy) intake so that you have the fuel you need to live your life.

One dietary adjustment that many women may make is increasing the amount of protein in their diets. Protein is a food fuel that helps us feel full and gives us the building blocks we need to maintain our bodies—our bones, muscles, skin, and blood. For example, after completing a brief dietary analysis, many women are surprised to find that they are not consuming the daily recommended amount of protein that they need. I encourage you to consider using a food journal or diary to see what kinds of foods you're eating and whether the variety and portions align with recommendations for your age and activity level. Perhaps the results will surprise you. There are plenty of excellent free tools, like the USDA MyPlate site, MyFitnessPal, and other health apps that can help you track food and liquid intake. I am not suggesting that you track every bite, but a short-term analysis of your current food and drink intake may help you to see the big picture and make changes if needed.

Our Relationship with Food

I am not a nutritionist, but I do know that our emotional relationship with food is one reason that people struggle with their nutritional choices. For some people, food is about energy; for others it is about celebration. Food can be comforting; it can be the enemy; it can be the last thing you want to prepare at the end of a long day. The prevalence of disordered eating and unhealthy relationships to food among middle-aged and older women is not well researched; however, bodily changes that naturally occur as women age can retrigger or ignite these issues. Eating disorders fall into one of three categories: bulimia nervosa (binging and purging), anorexia nervosa (severe food restriction and body image preoccupation), and binge eating (eating large amounts of food in secret). Common questions to consider regarding your relationship with food include: (1) How preoccupied are you with your body image as compared with other women you know? (2) If you could choose between living longer or attaining a "perfect weight," which would you choose? (3) Do you associate with people who spend a good deal of time talking about weight, dieting, and exercise? (4) Do you spend a lot of time thinking about what you eat and how much you exercise? (5) Do you practice eating habits that involve restricting food or eliminating certain foods from your diet? If your answers to these questions reflect a preoccupation with your weight and food that you believe is unhealthy, you may want to consider discussing this with a medical provider or counselor. Thinking about your body image, food, and weight occasionally is fine; the key here is how much headspace it's taking up. If these issues are something you think about once or twice a week and don't change how you feel about yourself or limit the activities that you do, then you likely have a healthier relationship with food.

Movement

A client of mine wanted to do an amazing, flash mob–style dance with her son at his wedding. Her face lit up as she talked about this idea; she knew the exact song to play, the outfit to wear, and she was working with her son to make it special. The idea was inspired by sweet moments they had spent together when he was a young child. One thing held her back: her stamina. My client was not as active as she had been before the onset of the pandemic. She felt shame and self-hatred about the way her body looked in clothes after gaining weight, she had trouble learning the dance moves, and she was winded after practice, all of which created doubts that her vision would reflect the reality of what she could do on the dance floor.

As we worked through her self-defeating beliefs, we also examined the values that drove her desire to enact this special moment. What she really valued and wanted to tap into was savoring the moment and being present at a truly joyous event; she also wanted to celebrate, with the same wild abandon, the way that she and her son did with their impromptu dance parties to Elvis songs. It was one of the ways that she and her son connected even through rough times, and she hoped that some version of this everyday joy would follow him into his new marriage.

Honestly, stories like this are one of the reasons I love my job; people are beautiful and amazing. What motivated my client was her desire to live this moment to the fullest. What our work became was a discussion of how living every moment to the fullest included movement and self-care so that she could physically do the things that she wanted to. The question was, what did physical activity look like for her? What can it look like for all of us? Sometimes the answers to our questions don't require radical solutions; they can mean capitalizing on what we already do. For example, a study published in the *Journal of Women Aging* sought to determine if women met the Centers for Disease Control and Prevention's guidelines for physical activity through leisure, household, and outdoor activities. Researchers found that when middle-aged women met the criteria for physical activities through such activities, they achieved better scores on overall physical activity than those who didn't (Schaal et al., 2016).

The more we broaden our definition of movement, the more opportunities we may find to see ourselves as active people. Self-talk that I heard from my client and from other women is, "Well, I'm not an athlete," or "I don't think of myself as a fitness person." I think physical activity can be too narrowly defined as the things you do when you go to a gym, and they're not. Movement is cleaning the house, working in the yard, cleaning your car, getting groceries, hauling kids and animals, and all of the other tasks that we do to keep our lives on track.

When my client and I talked about broadening her definition of movement to be more accepting and encompassing of what she already did while also acknowledging that there were some activities she could change or increase, her world opened a bit more. She saw the tasks that she did every day, like walking the family dog and her fifteen-minute walks at work, as contributions to her overall movement goals. One way that she gauged these activities' benefits was to purchase a pedometer to track her steps. This tool also provided her some indication of how limited her movement was over the course of the day. Her belief in wanting to live her life to the fullest was challenged when she realized that she was more physically passive than active. She slowly realigned her physical activity to reflect her beliefs and values. This is not a story of a couch person who becomes a marathon runner. Rather, this is a story of a woman who was winded at dance lessons and started a regular walking ritual at various times during the day (because small steps do add up) to become one of the most badass flash mob moms to celebrate her son's wedding. I'll never hear an Elvis song the same way again.

WHEN IT COMES TO PHYSICAL HEALTH, WISDOM IS MY VALUE

I have had several physical health curveballs thrown at me during the last five years, and negotiating them has made me reevaluate my values. What I value now is wisdom: my inner wisdom of knowing my body and what is right for me. My medical professionals don't live in my body, they don't know how it feels when something is off, and they don't know what it's like when everything feels fine in my body and then something goes catastrophically wrong. I do.

My beliefs about my inner wisdom must be flexible because it is fallible. There are times that medical and health experts give me information that feels counterintuitive, so I must balance listening to myself with the advice of people who have specialized training that I don't. I also believe that in using my wisdom I will find ways to manage my physical health that serves me well and leads me to the best possible life as I age. The boundaries that I try to maintain to preserve my physical health are to keep my doctor's appointments, to eat healthy and nutritious foods (more on my vices later), to get the sleep that I need, and to manage my inner critic. Just like you, I'm a work in progress, and my life experiences have pushed me to really think about what I value regarding my physical health, and those values run deep. As you reflect on the value you wrote at the beginning of the chapter, consider how your inner wisdom plays into your experience.

TELL ME WHAT YOU CAN DO, NOT WHAT YOU CAN'T DO

When I work with clients to set behavioral goals, I try to get them to think about how they can positively state their goals. We've likely all heard about "SMART" goals; the acronym stands for specific, measurable, achievable, realistic, timely. Relating SMART goals to physical health is particularly useful because it can give you very clear-cut, actionable tasks. But let's take it a step further: when making your goals, state them positively—tell yourself what you can do, not what you can't do. Stopping certain behaviors can be hard, like trying to quit smoking or drinking too much coffee (*she types while drinking her fifth cup of coffee today*). Instead, set yourself up for success by creating positively stated goals that meet the SMART criteria. For example, consider the following goals:

- I will stop drinking too much coffee every day.
- I will drink a maximum of three cups of coffee per day for the next two weeks.

My first goal wasn't very specific. I couldn't measure it because there wasn't really anything to achieve (what is too much coffee?). It wasn't realistic because I didn't have anything to compare it to nor was it timely. However, my second goal was very specific. I can measure it (three sad cups); it is achievable (three cups isn't no cups, which would be cruel); it's realistic (I'm not even cutting my consumption down by half); and it's timely (I'm doing it for two weeks before reevaluating). More importantly, I've told myself what I can do, not what I can't do. This goal aligns with my value of wisdom. What I know (and you do, too) is that drinking five cups of coffee over the course of the day is going to leave me feeling wired, which isn't a good idea if I want to rest. I believe in my inner wisdom, which tells me that the five-cups-of-coffee-a-day habit is not good for me. Creating this goal is a way to implement this value and belief by creating a boundary that I can work toward to embody my physical health value. With this in mind, what physical health goal do you want to create using the SMART criteria above?

My goal: _____

_____

Try implementing your goal over the next week and evaluate how it goes. If you find success, keep it going for another week. Maybe it will become a habit. If it doesn't work, go back to the SMART acronym and see if adjusting your goal will help.

SOME IS BETTER THAN NONE

We started this chapter by reviewing your values regarding physical health and the beliefs and boundaries that contribute to your value. I confess that as I wrote, I assumed that you—like me and other women I know—are not consistent about taking care of your physical body in ways that align with your values. We are all busy, and our ability to consistently take care of our physical health is the first thing we tend to drop when life gets busy. I know that for me, when my movement, nutritional intake, and sleep start to become less of a priority, then my shame and inner critic start getting loud and make it challenging for me to love myself. Here's what I must remember, and what I want you to remember: *some is better than none.*

This is a mantra that I say to myself when I think that I haven't done "enough" to take care of my physical body. Yes, I ate ice cream for dinner, and I ate a salad with protein for lunch. Yes, I missed my one-hour yoga class, and I made time for a twenty-minute walk at work. Yes, I stayed up too late watching the last episode of my new favorite show, and I put on a twenty-minute timer so I could take a quick rest break in the afternoon to refresh. There is no such thing as perfection, and life gives us too many opportunities and curveballs to do all the physical health things every day. But do some and see where it leads you. Because you will feel better doing some than you will if you do none.

CHAPTER FIVE

APPEARANCE

What no one told me about midlife is that my face was going to break out like it was the second coming of my early teenage years. Scratch that—it was worse than my teen years: I had clear skin when I look back at pictures. After struggling for months, trying new serums, visiting an esthetician for facials, and bemoaning my erupting skin, I finally had an appointment with my dermatologist for my yearly checkup.

If you've ever been to a dermatologist, you know that they get excessively close to your skin to look at all defects there may be. They take a magnifier to look at moles and skin anomalies, make "hmmmm" sounds when they see something they have mixed emotions about, and look at portions of your body you wouldn't have thought were important to study because they typically don't see a lot of sun (unless you're a nudist, in which case you *should* have every crevice examined).

My dermatologist made a sympathetic mew and said, "Yes, you have a lot of comedones; we definitely should look into this." Comedone is the fancy medical term for zits. Acne at any age messes with your self-confidence, and I am no different. I had been slathering concealer and base onto my face in unheard-of ways for several months, so the hope for a fix was almost too much. Then came the punchline from my doctor: "The good thing is the medicine I'm going to give you should also help with all the lines on your face. It's kind of like getting two for one; it should help with the acne and with those age lines you have that are really starting to show."

I mean, *wow*. Clearly, I didn't come here for a pep talk, now did I? There is something demoralizing about a thirtysomething practitioner with glowing skin and access to cutting-edge products and technology looking at you with some mixture of sympathy and savior complex. Yes, I'm fully aware that I'm living at the intersection between acne and aging; I've seen mirrors. This experience was quite a wake-up call about the difference between how I see myself (in the mirror) and how other people see me. Some days, on the inside, I still feel like I'm seventeen, twenty-five, thirty-seven, but on the outside, the midyears show on my body and my face. How we look and present to the world is an important part of our identity, and yet if we say that out loud, we may be perceived as shallow, vain, or narcissistic. It's funny to think that we live in a culture in which maintaining youth is a top priority, yet if we express feelings about how we are physically showing signs of aging, we may experience judgment. This conundrum makes this chapter hard to write; articulating the experiences of many women while battling my own inner critic who keeps saying, "You're not supposed to admit to this because it makes you appear vain," is complicated. If you're like me, fighting internalized messages may be part of your process as you read this chapter.

Research suggests that individuals are perceived as less attractive as they start to look older (Samson et al., 2010). In my literature review before writing this chapter, I found an article about perceptions of women who engage in facial age concealment. Researchers found that women tend to judge other women most harshly for using antiaging treatments, particularly if the treatments were used to gain better employment or a romantic partner (Childs & Jones, 2023). In this study, "age concealment" methods ranged from using therapeutic red light (passive treatment) to skin injectables (invasive treatment). Although not all of us use antiaging treatments, the changes in our faces and bodies may lead us to judge ourselves; knowing that research shows that others may be judging us as well is another bitter pill to swallow.

INTERNAL VALIDATION

Years ago, during the great ashram excursion, I was sitting in silence (I wore a badge with my name that said I was practicing silence) when a very good-looking guy joined me at my table. He introduced himself and told me that he had just arrived at the ashram and would be working there in exchange for room and board. He needed to leave his hometown and start over. He then proceeded to tell me his life story, mixed in with flirting. I guess if 90 percent of communication is nonverbal, then silence isn't an obstacle. And he was *good-looking*. He said lovely things, telling me all the things a girl wants to hear about herself. Then came the line that ended it all: "You're a really good listener." *Dude, I'm in silence, of course, I'm a good listener.*

This was a point in my life when I felt emotionally low. I had sought refuge and restoration in a mountain retreat to get my life back on track, and here was temptation staring me right in the face, with a very charming smile. I smiled back, picked up my food tray, and walked back to my room. My immediate thought when he started flirting was, "Oh thank goodness, I've still got it." Because we all have times in our lives when we want to feel desirable, and at this time in my life, when I could see my face and body changing, I wasn't feeling great about myself. My confidence in myself was low, and if I'd stayed and continued to (nonverbally) flirt or do whatever might have happened in that interaction, then I still would have been seeking external validation about how I felt about myself. I walked away because I had to rely on myself to internally validate how I felt about my appearance and desirability. What I mean by internal validation is accepting my thoughts and feelings about myself as my truth and living within that truth.

Our worth isn't dictated by our appearance, and yet we are immersed in a culture that says women's worth is very much dictated by our appearance. What are we to do with those messages as we age? Because we will age, and as our elders say, "It's better than the alternative," which is to be dead. We need to accept the fact that our appearance will change and internally validate ourselves regarding how we look and carry ourselves through midlife and beyond. You may choose to go with the flow, fight it, or land somewhere in between—no matter your path, change is happening. A bigger question is, how can you love and accept these changes as positive and life-affirming rather than as loss? Let's talk about how we can do it within our values and meet reality on our terms.

REFLECTION QUESTIONS

How did you perceive older women when you were younger? As a girl and young adult, I often thought of the women who are my current age as mature. These early memories can provide a template for our beliefs about getting older.

- What values do you hold about your appearance?
- How much of a role does your appearance play in the overall package that is you?
- What messages did you receive about being a woman and how your body would change as you aged?
- Were they positive or negative messages?
- What changes in your appearance make you happy and proud?

THE SCIENCE OF AGING AND THE IMPACT ON OUR APPEARANCE

Examining medical and scientific research is the best way to explain the aging process in-depth. Science shows that menopause creates the biggest shift in aging in women and a big impact on our appearance. When we move through menopause, our bodies reduce the production of sex hormones (as much as 80% less estrogen, for example), and around the same time, we also begin losing collagen in our skin. Men tend to have more gradual hormonal declines and lose collagen throughout their lifespans, whereas women tend to have more dramatic shifts in these two areas during and after menopause. These biological differences may be why people perceive that men age more gradually, whereas women may experience more dramatic shifts in their looks as they get older.

So what are the specific impacts of sex hormone shifts and collagen, and how do these affect our appearance? Our two main sex hormones are androgen and estrogen. Lessening androgen levels can cause additional loss of estrogen, which is women's main sex hormone. The impact of lower androgen levels can include weight gain, impairment in sexual functioning, loss of bone density, lessening physical functioning (ability to gain muscle mass), emotional changes, and cognitive changes. Of these, changes in weight, lessening physical functioning, and emotional changes can have the biggest impact on our appearance (Rubinstein & Foster, 2013).

The reduced production of estrogen impacts how your body uses fats and carbohydrates, your ability to recover from injuries, inflammatory responses in your body, and changes in muscle strength. These changes can result in body weight fluctuations and impact your ability to recover from physical activity and to maintain and build muscle tone in your body. Estrogen also influences general mood and emotions, which also can be reflected in your appearance. Pain, discomfort, and distress have an embodied look that can impact how you carry yourself and is reflected in your face. Lower estrogen also can affect hair, which can become thinner and grow more slowly.

Finally, collagen is a protein found in skin and connective tissue that makes your skin look elastic and gives it the ability to "bounce back." To me, one of the best measures of collagen loss is the evidence of "pillow face" in the morning. When I was young, the pillow creases in my face from sleep were gone by the time I brushed my teeth in the morning. Now I'm staring at them during my morning commute a good two hours after I've woken up and wondering when they'll finally be gone for the day. Since your skin covers your entire body, it's worth noting that what's happening on your face is also happening all over your body. With skin, it's not only collagen loss that impacts our appearance, but also sun exposure/skin damage, how hydrated or dry our skin is, and how thin our skin is on certain parts of our bodies (neck, elbows, knees, eyes) that contribute to how we look to ourselves and others.

Supernormal Stimuli

For me, knowledge is power, so I want to share something with you that changed my perspective about how I'm aging. It relates to media and something called supernormal stimuli, which are artificial stimuli that can trigger a stronger reaction than the one for which the instinct evolved (Barrett, 2016). Supernormal stimuli were first discovered in an experiment in which birds were exposed to their natural eggs and to larger fake eggs. Scientists found again and again that birds and other species gravitated toward protecting and nurturing larger fake eggs rather than the natural ones. The animal's internalized instinct is to respond to an egg, but when presented with a bigger and better "egg," its instinct elicited a stronger response than would naturally occur, and it gravitated toward the large fake egg.

An example of supernormal stimuli in the human realm is pornography. Some versions of pornography give the viewer an exaggerated experience of sexual encounters (for example, larger than typical breasts or penises). After repeated watching and over time, viewers can become less sexually responsive to normal stimuli in favor of the supernormal stimuli (which may not be attainable in real life). Other examples of supernormal stimuli in our lives include hyperpalatable foods (formerly known as "junk" food) or media usage. Think about our exposure to popular media today through television, movies, and social media. These are all places in which photo filters and artificial intelligence (AI) are used to make individuals look more attractive than they may be in real life. You may recall that Julia Roberts had a body double for the legs in the movie poster for *Pretty Woman*. The phenomenon of attempting to make people (women) look "better" through supernormal stimuli isn't new.

Applying the idea of supernormal stimuli to aging, images of younger women or AI-enhanced images of women may be misrepresented as those of older age groups in the media. This "trick" isn't new, but its ubiquity—it pervades our culture to such an extent that it can be difficult to tell what's real and what's not—is more recent. People can access image-editing tools easily with cell phones. This exposes us to unrealistic messages about appearance and aging through a filtered lens or AI generation, and the consequences can be our self-esteem and feelings of self-worth. We may start to question why our fifty-one-year-old self looks so different from the (enhanced) fifty-one-year-old in the media, which may trigger negative self-talk. Research supports this. A study published in 2024 found that photo editing has negative effects on perceived physical appearance and mood (Wolfe & Yakabovits, 2024). Knowing the difference between what is real and fake is important in maintaining realistic expectations for ourselves as we move through life stages. Knowing how biology and technology impact our experience of aging is important as we negotiate changes in our appearance. Next, let's explore how we come to a greater realization about these changes.

STAGES OF REALIZATION

I remember being young and thinking that I couldn't wait to get older, not just because of the privileges that came with age (driving looked pretty good), but also because I would look older and less like a child. To give some context, I am the youngest in my family, and *everyone* looked older, seemed to have more freedom, and was certainly way cooler than I. Looking back, I know this is an illusion. But I remember fantasizing about what it would be like to look older. I used to suck my cheeks in to see what I'd look like without my baby face (nowadays they perform "buccal fat removal" to make cheekbones more prominent), contort myself to make my neck look wrinkly, and try to figure out where the lines in my face would be when I got older. (At the dermatologist's office, an advertisement stated that to ward off signs of aging, you should avoid repetitive motions with your face—my teachers were right, my face *will* freeze in that expression.)

Then I got older, went off to college, and started living my life. I caught up with the people around me, I looked older, and I got the privileges and responsibilities that come with adulthood. There are days when I do feel a little bit cool for all that I've accomplished. But here's the thing about working on a college campus like I do—every fall a fresh batch of eighteen-year-olds shows up to remind me that I have achieved what I wanted all those years ago: I do look older, and time is marching all over my face and my body.

My early realizations that I was starting to look older began gradually, and there were changes that I was fine with, things like gray hairs and laugh lines. These are easy to cover up with hair dye or the careful application of makeup to avoid accentuating the lines (oh, the early lines were minimal—a preview of coming attractions). These signs started showing in my thirties, so they didn't seem like that big of a deal, more of a rite of passage and a sign that I was becoming a "real" adult. I saw the same things happening in the faces of my friends who were on their life journeys of coupling, having kids, building careers, and creating their homes; these signs were validation of where we were in our lives.

But then things start to get more real, and it becomes harder to deny that aging is happening to you, and it is going to impact how you look and present to the world. For me, this wasn't something that started with my face; rather, it began with my foot. I've already discussed my arthritic feet in chapter 4, which changed how I exercise and ultimately how I saw myself as a "healthy" person. One of the things that I did as a reaction to this diagnosis was to stop exercising for a while, which made me feel terrible and hurt my body. Fast-forward to trying to get into a lower-impact sport, so I decide to take swimming lessons at my local Y. My swimming instructor was so good at coaching me through strokes, but the coup de grâce (or death blow for those of us who don't speak *français*) was when she told me that I would need to take it slow and that although I could build my stamina, because of my age, my lung capacity would not reach the levels it had when I was younger.

I got it; I wasn't going to be Michael Phelps at the end of my lesson, but couldn't I aim for Dara Torres? She didn't quit participating in the Olympics until she was in her forties. Sadly, acceptance means that I will also not be Dara Torres by the time I'm out of my forties; that ship has sailed. But these experiences catalyzed my hard look at where I was in my life—and that was in the middle of it. I spoke with a friend about this at a conference weeks later and she laughed because she had done her makeup in the magnified hotel mirror. I remember her saying, "Yeah, hello forty-three—magnified times ten—that's the greeting I got this morning."

Her comment prompted me to take a gander at my hotel mirror, and *whoa!* I took a (literal) hard look at myself and realized that there wasn't room for denial, that the changes in my appearance—on my face and in my body—weren't going away, they were here to stay, and they were also taking up residence and making themselves comfortable. I have a permanent frown line between my eyes, the dimple lines in my cheeks don't bounce back, don't get me started on the cellulite, and I recently discovered that what I thought were freckles on my hands are *age spots*.

These cumulative experiences and reflections that we have with friends bring home a truth that many of us try to resist. We are getting older, our appearance is changing, and the way that other people relate to us also changes because we look older. It can cause us to reflect about how aging impacts how others see us and how we see ourselves. Early experiences of others treating you differently as you age and as your appearance changes can seem like one-offs, but as they increase in frequency, this can reinforce how your worth may be changing in society. Examples of being treated differently can include being dismissed or ignored in favor of younger or more attractive women, being treated deferentially to the point of condescension, or being told you "look good for a lady your age." Managing how others treat us based on our appearance can range from acceptance to resistance to outright denial. To be sure, being treated differently based on our aging looks can take a toll, and these experiences can weigh us down and take up our headspace from time to time.

In my work with women for whom it did take up a lot of headspace, they spent a lot of time worrying about how others would perceive them as they aged, how desired they would be, and where their power would come from if their looks weren't something that they had to rely on. Worrying took away their happiness, robbed them of embracing all the wonderful qualities they possess beyond their appearance, and negated the fact that they were very attractive—albeit in older bodies. I can't say with certainty that men don't have to manage these same issues as they age, but I must believe that their experiences are very different than women's. It's important to highlight and openly acknowledge that we live in a society that tells women that part of their worth is linked to their overall appearance. The fallacy of this standard is that aging is inevitable, and no matter how a woman tries to resist it, her physical appearance changes as she gets older.

Women fall along a spectrum. Some read this chapter and see their changing appearance as a nonevent; for others it is a passing thought, but there are more pressing things to focus on. Aging and appearance may be a call to arms to "age gracefully" but not to "look like my mother," whereas for some it is a daily review and revision of how they can maintain or fix their appearance to look younger than they are. Falling somewhere along this spectrum is acceptable so long as it feels healthy to you.

When I was doing my yoga teacher training in 2015, I read an article about Seane Corn featured in *Yoga Journal*. Ms. Corn, a well-known yoga teacher and activist, discussed how her life was changing now that she was turning fifty. The spirit of one of her quotes has stuck with me all these years, because she mentioned that part of turning fifty was about accepting the next phase of her life and the loss of her beauty. At the time I didn't understand what she was talking about, and at this stage of my life, I find it very refreshing that she said this in her interview. Openly acknowledging her appearance as a part of her transition into midlife and beyond—particularly as someone who is perceived as a highly trained yogi and who transcends material concerns—was powerful, normalizing, and humanizing. But that doesn't mean that accepting one's changing appearance always happens gracefully or willingly.

Denial and Rejection

We can certainly try to resist or deny the reflection in the mirror and pretend that we're not looking any older, but to do this denies the path that our lives are taking. Whether it is one specific event that drew your attention to the changes in your appearance or several cumulative ones, at some point you will see that you don't look the same as you did in those pictures of yourself from fifteen years ago. Couple this realization with the fact that even with modern innovations in face and body cream, makeup, and more invasive procedures, some things are not fixable, no matter how much you may wish things to be different.

Our changing body and appearance offer us an opportunity to embrace the fact that there are aspects of the aging process that make us better than we were before. I harken back to the "refined" version of who we are. The older I get, the more I appreciate that my mannerisms, expressions, and expression lines remind me of people I've loved and lost. As I age, resemblances, either physical or behavioral, become more entrenched—like a time machine that merges the past with the present. I don't believe this is limited to biology; I think it can be about emotions and behaviors that we've picked up from the important nonbiological people in our lives, and I find those reminders just as precious as I get older.

No matter where you are in the spectrum of acceptance, a catalyst will push you to the insight that you will never look any younger than you look today (that's called reality and the space-time continuum). You can choose to deny this reality, but denial won't change the fact. However, there are steps we can take to potentially preserve how we appear to ourselves and others, ranging from more mainstream to unusual. A mainstream example might be using sunscreen, which protects our skin from the sun's harmful rays, helping prevent cancer and premature skin aging. This is a more "socially acceptable" intervention that most people can support. An example of something more unusual might be getting a platelet-rich plasma facial (PRP), known as the "vampire facial."

This is a medical procedure in which a patient's blood is taken and put through a centrifuge to isolate the PRP and then the person's face is microneedled and spread with the plasma to promote collagen growth. PRP also is used in other medical procedures, such as injections into the joints for orthopedic issues, which was the original intention of the intervention. I have a friend who had a PRP and loved it; she thought it improved her skin health and helped lessen the appearance of wrinkles and scars. I don't like giving blood *at all*, so the thought of smearing my plasma all over my face after microinjections makes me nervous. And if you want to try it, then do it, girl! We may try these interventions because they give us a sense of control over how we age, which is inherently out of our control.

All of this brings me back to when I was younger and I was *dying* to get older, get my period, and grow up. I remember reading the scene in Judy Blume's book *Are You There God? It's Me, Margaret*, where the girls get together to do their bust-building exercises: "I must, I must, I must increase my bust." I remember laughing with my friends as we talked about that scene and then tried to reenact it in the hopes that we could grow our busts too! And now here we are, trying to slow the clock down rather than speed it up, which will have as much impact as that silly exercise did, although it helps to feel as if we have some sense of control over the process. And isn't that what we're all looking for—a sense of control in our lives when we have very few ways to control the changes that we're going through?

Mourning versus Embracing

In 2021 Justine Bateman authored a book called *Face: One Square Foot of Skin*. It's a series of short stories that she wrote about women at different ages and stages of their lives that highlights the importance of women aging on their terms and not listening to the messages promoted ubiquitously in media and culture that women should "fix" or "change" their faces and bodies as they age to meet a status quo. What is ingenious about her book is that she asks her readers to consider how they came to the place where they believed that how they looked wasn't "okay" or acceptable in some way. This is a thought-provoking question, particularly because, even after writing this chapter, I haven't found a good answer to that very question. I wonder if you feel the same way. It feels as though the expectation for preserving my appearance has always been with me. If I were to shake off this expectation and reject it as not my own because I don't think I was born thinking this, how might my life look different? If you shook off these same expectations, how might your life look different?

Questioning internalized expectations makes me think about a shopping trip that I took with my mother when she was in her late forties or early fifties. She was shopping for a dress for some event, and we went through several different styles and sizes to see if she could find something that worked. Fashions for women in her age group in the late 1990s and early 2000s were not exactly kind. My mother is petite, and at that time finding a wide variety of petite clothing was challenging. After trying on yet another dress, I asked her how she liked it. We were both feeling tired and discouraged at this point, and I remember her saying, "I feel fat and middle-aged." What she didn't say, but I heard in my heart, is that she felt disempowered, unsure of her looks and place in the world as a woman, and her self-judgment was through the roof. I hate that she felt that way because my mother is a strong, tough, and independent woman; at no point in my life have I seen her any other way. It wasn't her vulnerability that disarmed me, it was the fact that this shopping expedition crystallized the thoughts and feelings she was having about herself in her midlife.

The lesson I take from this is that no matter who we are—from famous actresses to average women—it can be shocking to realize that we are not immune to the changes that middle age brings to our appearance and feelings about our self-worth. We tend to feel a loss because we may perceive that these changes are shameful, less desirable, or have forever changed the internalized image of whom we believed we were during early stages of our lives. I think it's fair to say that this phenomenon is more specific to women since we live in a culture in which much of women's currency is predicated on their physical appearance. The point here is that you aren't shallow or bad if you mourn your appearance and its natural changes. What you do with your mourning is important. If it becomes a central focus, if you get stuck thinking about these changes, or if you engage in unhealthy behaviors like sabotaging younger women because you perceive them as a threat, there could be more there to explore. Sorrow is one thing, but getting stuck in sorrow is giving in to the social convention that you are only as important as how you look; that is simply not true.

So, after all of this, what does it mean to embrace your midlife appearance? First, we are not alone in these changes, and even supermodels don't look like supermodels after time has passed. One example of this in celebrity news is the photos of Pamela Anderson attending Paris Fashion Week in 2023. She made appearances without makeup and was quoted as saying, "I'm not trying to be the prettiest girl in the room. I feel like it's just freedom. It's release." Anderson went on to say that she believes that it's her responsibility to model age and self-acceptance at a time when these are not the norms for women (Clack, 2023).

Ms. Anderson's sentiment is true. You are more than how you look in this world; you are the culmination of your experiences, relationships, and work that has brought you to the place where you are in your life. If we start to look at these changes with more curiosity than fear or anger, what might be revealed to us? It could be the faces of our grandparents; it could be lines that show our resilience through tough times and laugh lines that remind us that we enjoyed easier times. It could be the stretch marks that you earned when you brought your babies into the world and the veined, age-spotted hands that work hard to care for others. Our appearance weathers like a pair of jeans because we are weathering the journey of life; the evidence that shows in our bodies and faces is further proof of our lives. As we age and it shows in our appearance, we are further refined and closer to the true architecture of our souls. And who doesn't want their true soul to shine through?

More defiant confrontations of the women and aging trope are found in early 2023, when Madonna was the subject of scrutiny at awards shows, which led to her making the statement, "I have never apologized for any of the creative choices I have made nor the way that

I look or dress and I'm not going to start. I have been degraded by the media since the beginning of my career, but I understand that this is all a test, and I am happy to do the trailblazing so that all the women behind me can have an easier time in the years to come" (Yamada, 2023). Whether or not you agree with the Material Girl's choices, her power move of not backing down from her choices related to her appearance is one that we can all identify with.

Empowerment

Empowerment means that we have the authority to do what we think is best for ourselves. Acceptance is more about something being satisfactory or adequate. I think that first accepting our changing appearance is an important part of the aging process, but I believe that feeling empowered by these changes is worth striving for. At this point in our lives, our bodies have carried us (literally) through half a lifetime—what an accomplishment! Those years likely have been filled with both good and bad times, and we are showing signs of this half of a lifetime lived. I remember when I was going through puberty and into early adulthood as a young woman. Self-acceptance and body satisfaction were important messages that I received from the adults around me. I would be asked questions like, "What do you love about your body? What do you love about the way that you look?" As a beginning counselor, I asked these same questions to the young women that I worked with in a therapeutic group focused on building body positivity as a part of good mental health practices. Why do we stop reinforcing this self-acceptance as we age?

As a woman in midlife, there are things about my appearance that I love. I love that when I smile, my dimples are deeper than ever before. I love that my freckles still show how much I enjoy the sun on my face. I love that my body is strong, and I can go for long walks and lift weights, even if my stamina is not quite what it was twenty years ago. I love that my boobs are healthy and still attached to me, because it was questionable there for a minute.

At this stage, I am grateful to be here and to be able to plan the next part of my life. Although my appearance is an important part of the package that is me, it is a fraction of all that I am. I hope that as you have read through this chapter you have found clarity about how you perceive your appearance. Although we may certainly give the changes in our appearance some attention, we know that what we love about our appearance and ourselves far outweighs the things that may trouble us (I'm talking to you, saggy neck). As you think about your aging appearance, try these reflections and exercises to examine your journey toward acceptance and empowerment.

AGING AND APPEARANCE EXERCISE

Thinking back to a question earlier in this chapter about realistic expectations regarding appearance and aging and realistic role models in our lives led me to create this exercise. I hope you find some inspiration in it as well. Reflect on your thoughts about aging by answering the questions below.

If I didn't have a personal expectation to preserve my appearance, what might be different in my life? _____

_____

Who are the women in my life that I want to emulate as I move into midlife and beyond? _____

_____

What wisdom can I learn from them about my aging appearance? _____

_____

_____

How am I empowered to love my changing appearance and body as I age?

_____

_____

Some sample answers to these questions follow.

If I didn't have a personal expectation to preserve my appearance, what might be different in my life? *I would spend a lot less time, energy, and money on skincare products. I would care for my body without getting wrapped up in fads.*

Who are the women in my life that I want to emulate as I move into midlife and beyond? *My friend Leslie who is seventy and one of the most fun, spontaneous, and lively women I know.*

What wisdom can I learn from them about my aging appearance? *Leslie is honest about how she's struggled with her changing appearance; she talks me through her journey by living her biggest, healthiest life by taking care of her body, with no apologies to anyone.*

How am I empowered to love my changing appearance and body as I age? *I am empowered to see my parents' faces in my own. I feel and look strong and healthy, which is so important to me and aligns with my values.*

REFLECTION QUESTIONS

- What do you love about your appearance and your body?
- How can you feel good in the body/skin that you're in?
- How are you aging in line with your values?

Aging and our appearance deserve to be discussed openly, honestly, and without judgment or shame. As we move into our midlife, we discover that change is happening, and our evolving looks do not have to take center stage in our identity as women. I know I've used famous women as examples throughout this chapter, but our mothers, aunts, and best friends are not available for public scrutiny. I'm glad about that—the public can be brutal. Because these famous women navigate the constant recording of their changing appearance in the public eye, I think they are good examples demonstrating how we all can embrace our physical evolution in midlife. I think this quote from Regina King sums it up best, "I feel like I'm so much more interesting now, as a soon-to-be-50-year-old woman, than I was at 25. I can bring so much more to the table. You may not have the stamina that you had at 25, but what you know now? So much better" (Marks, 2021).

I recently reread Nora Ephron's book *I Feel Bad about My Neck and Other Thoughts on Being a Woman* (2008), which is a superbly funny account of aging. In it, she laments that one of her regrets in life is that she didn't spend more time admiring her neck before it began to sag and age. This is a smart, funny, talented woman speaking the truth about the natural progression of our lives and our appearance. It's validating to know that other talented women are honest about such a sensitive subject. Although we must ultimately be able to internally validate how we feel about our appearance as we age, it can be important to have people with whom we talk and share experiences regarding how we look in midlife and as we continue to evolve and change. I hope that we can inspire the next generation of ladies who are aging behind us that although things do inevitably change, embracing our looks and owning our inherent beauty is an important part of midlife and beyond.

We are the sum of our parts, appearance included. This can be a big or small part of how you see yourself, but like our discussion about the architecture of the soul, finding and refining your place in midlife won't necessarily center on your appearance. Likely it centers more on your relationship. This brings us to love, which reveals our beauty through how well we love and are loved. Let's find out how big the world of love can be.

CHAPTER SIX

INTIMATE RELATIONSHIPS

A memory circles my mind occasionally that feels as real to me now as it did thirty years ago. My dad and I are coming home after a family trip. It's night and he's driving, and we're almost home. I can remember the stretch of I-20 we're on, that feeling of exhaustion from being in the car for seven hours and the relief that we're almost home after a long day. He must have been tired because he was trying to find something to listen to on the radio to keep him awake. Suddenly the song "Moon River" plays on the radio, and he stops fiddling and we listen as it begins. *"Moon River, wider than a mile, I'm crossing you in style someday."*

Of course, I'd heard the *Breakfast at Tiffany's* version, but something about the quiet of the car and the sounds of the song as it was performed in my father's youth, changed the tone of the ride. I remember looking at him driving in the darkness and feeling a profound sense of peace and safety. Hands on the wheel (at two and ten), he was looking straight ahead, lost in his own thoughts. I wonder what he was thinking. I look back on that memory and hear the song again, *"two drifters, off to see the world, there's such a lot of world to see."*

We were in such different places, as parents and children are, my dad in the middle of his life, not very far from where I am now. And me, a girl with everything ahead of her, full of the natural angst that comes from being young and both sure and unsure. Yet we were in the exact same place, two people forever linked by our familial bond and our relationship, which was essential to each of us and allowed us to be our true selves. My father and I didn't have a perfect relationship; we could be more similar than different, which led to conflict. But he tried to understand me, and as I got older, we grew into an adult relationship that was built on mutual understanding, appreciation, and love. We had fascinating conversations; he had done so many things in his life. He was intrigued by and curious about the world, and this trait could be both interesting and exasperating.

But at that moment, with the moonlight shining in the car windows and this song guiding us a few miles closer to home, neither of us could know what our relationship would become. The song itself is a metaphor for romantic love, with a bittersweet melody that guides the listener through the hope and heartbreak that can result from relationships. What I hear every time my heart is broken is the memory of my father's voice, "Oh, Elizabeth, this too shall pass." His presence is remarkably present in my life, even though he is gone. What he taught me about love, about trying to be the best version of myself for my relationships, endures. Although love can sometimes mean tumult, the overarching feeling can be safety and acceptance. That is powerful. I reach back to that moment of us riding in the car together because it reminds me of one of the most profound gifts of love that I was given. I grieve for him because grief is part of love; it reminds me of how important love is. In our lives we search for love and connection with the people closest to us. Sometimes we get it right and sometimes we don't, and yet we keep trying. Love, in its many forms, is a powerful and essential part of our existence that we reach for because it is how we find meaning. That it can feel elusive and confusing is why we struggle with it. And yet, if we're lucky, we will find it in the most unexpected places. *"We're after the same rainbow's end, waitin' 'round the bend, my huckleberry friend . . ."*

LOVE AND INTIMATE RELATIONSHIPS

When we talk about intimate relationships, people often default to sexual relationships, which is a type of intimacy but not the only kind. Intimacy is defined as "something of a personal or private nature, belonging to or characterizing one's deepest nature," according to Merriam-Webster. One word that comes up when I think of intimacy is "vulnerability," because if you have a close personal relationship with someone with whom you share your deepest self, then it means that you have shared with them private thoughts and feelings that you don't share with the outside world. It also means that you've built the relationship over time, which enables the person to know you well enough to read you and intuit what you may be feeling in certain situations. To build intimacy, reciprocity between the two people is necessary; the vulnerability is mutual.

Current statistics show that marriage and divorce rates have declined in the last decade, meaning that fewer people are getting married and fewer people are getting divorced (US Census Bureau, 2020). These numbers don't include individuals who are in partnerships, such as cohabitants, but who are not married. Additionally, the number of people who have never been married has also risen in the last decade, meaning that a greater percentage of the population, across all age groups and genders, are not marrying at previous rates. At any given point in a woman's life, she may be without a romantic partner. This can be by choice or due to divorce or separation, death, or some other reason. In the United States, between 17 and 20 percent of women report being divorced during their midlife years and between 1 and 8 percent report being widowed during their midlife years. Does this mean that if you don't have a romantic partner, you don't have intimate relationships? Absolutely not! In this chapter we discuss the different types of love that are the hallmarks of intimate relationships, how to identify who you have intimate relationships with (your inner circle), and how you show them love and care. We also use tools to identify toxicity in relationships and exercises to clarify the health of your most important relationships.

THE MANY TYPES OF LOVE

Romantic love tends to get most people's attention. In the abstract, it is ideal, a feeling to seek out, and it is "terrible" if we don't have it. Writers and artists extol the virtues of romantic love in their works, and it permeates popular culture through songs, movies, and books across cultures and time. The idea of romantic love is thought to have first originated in the late eighteenth century in France with the rise of what was referred to as "courtly love." In our lives, love takes many forms, and its meanings are complex and multilayered. In this section, we briefly look at eight of the different types of love defined by the Greeks: eros, *ludus*, mania, *philia*, storge, agape, *pragma*, and *philautia*.

- *Eros* is defined as romantic love and is associated with sexuality and physical desire. This type of love can be challenging to sustain and is what people often seek to maintain within their relationships.
- *Ludus* is "playful love," which is linked with feelings of infatuation. It may or may not develop into eros. The feelings of butterflies in your stomach, giddiness, and anticipation that characterize a new relationship are examples of how someone may feel when they are in ludus.
- *Mania*, or obsessive love, is the type of love that can lead to jealousy, irrational decision making, and anger. This type of love can be frightening and abusive; it is also associated with extreme passion, which may be desired by some.
- *Philia*, or affectionate love, is the type of love individuals feel for friends or people who are close to them. It is characterized as a love between equals and was prized by the Greeks as love in its highest form, even more sought after than romantic love.
- *Storge* is the love felt between parents and children or family members. It is characterized by a strong bond or feelings of kinship that develops over time. This term is typically defined by biological relationships, but given the importance of families of choice in our culture, I believe the definition can include any type of family.
- *Agape* is unconditional, altruistic, and selfless love. This type of love has been characterized as a spiritual type of love that few can attain. In Christianity, it is akin to the sacrifice that Jesus made for humanity. When I think of this love, I am reminded of the parents I have seen caring for their adult children who are developmentally delayed and dependent on them. Without fanfare or complaint, this love demonstrates the highest form of care for another.
- *Pragma* is referred to as enduring love, which is considered by some to be the opposite of eros. *Pragma* love takes time to mature and develop. Examples include couples or friends who have been together or known each other for a long time and still find joy and contentment in each other's company.

- *Philautia* is what we refer to as self-love and is characterized as a necessary element to keep ourselves healthy and whole; it is how we regard ourselves and engage in self-care to maintain a positive sense of self-regard. Taken too far, it can be seen as selfish, egocentric, or narcissistic. In practice, this type of love might be expressed through the healthy use of boundaries.

Here's what I appreciate about this list: there's plenty of love to go around. When we broaden our view of love and are more inclusive about how we can experience it, we may find that we are surrounded by more than we realize. Intimacy is part of the experience of love, and we can share intimacy with ourselves, our parents, caregivers, siblings, family, friends, coworkers, romantic partners, children, and, in some cases, pets. By widening our perspective about what intimacy is and engaging with others to share deeply personal moments, I think we may find that our lives are much richer and less lonely than they may sometimes feel.

WHO IS IN YOUR INNER CIRCLE?

When I work with women on their relationships, I often ask them to imagine who is in their inner circle. The people in the inner circle aren't necessarily all the same people in your social circle. Instead, they are the few with whom you are your most vulnerable. This doesn't mean that the relationships with people in your inner circle are the smoothest, easiest, or healthiest ones. Instead, these can be some of our most challenging relationships—and our most important ones. Take a moment and reflect on who is in your inner circle.

It can be helpful to think about this idea as an actual circle. Using figure 6.1, complete your own inner circle by adding the names of the people in your life in the circle. The smallest circle is your inner circle, or the people with whom you have the most intimate relationships. The middle circle includes the people with whom you're socially close to. The largest circle is for the people in your life with whom you have relationships that aren't as close as your social or intimate relationships.

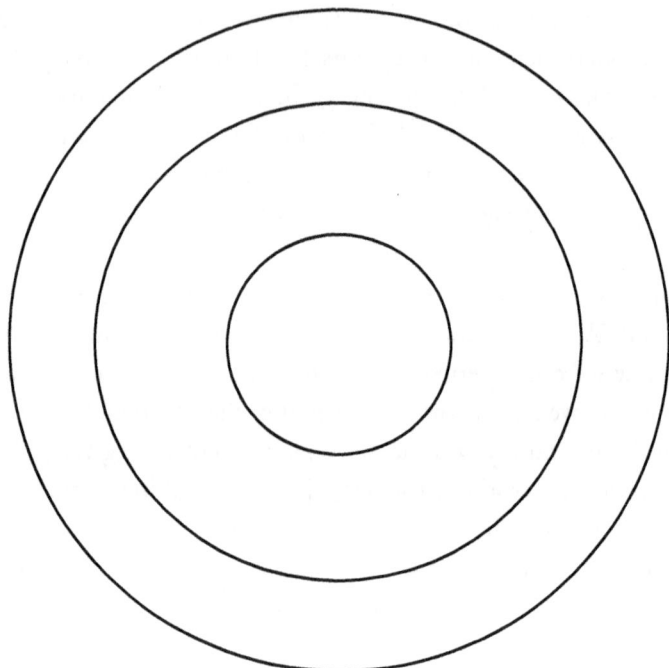

Figure 6.1. Your Inner Circle

This exercise becomes challenging for women when they reflect on the important people in their lives and realize that they may be more vulnerable with people whom they wouldn't consciously include in their inner circle, such as coworkers. Conversely, after an internal inventory, some women may discover that they feel less close to people whom they might have included in the inner circle without reflection, such as their spouse or a sibling. I see this scenario play out most often in marriages and partnerships, and it can be a wake-up call.

Reaching back to the values sort in chapter 2, what values did you pick that relate to intimate relationships? What are the beliefs and boundaries that align with these values? Taking this reflection a step further, also consider how people in your life might demonstrate this value to you and how you demonstrate the value back to them. Table 6.1 gives you an example to help guide your reflection.

Table 6.1. Sample Reflection

Value	Belief	Boundary	Person	Demonstration
Honesty	Telling the truth is part of showing trust.	When sharing honest feedback (good or bad) it should be delivered in a way that the person can hear.	Partner	• I demonstrate honesty to my partner by giving them feedback about how I worry about their health and encourage them to seek treatment when they need it. • My partner demonstrates honesty to me by giving me feedback about my work habits that can impact our time together.
Kindness	Showing kindness to important people in my life is one of the ways I show love and care.	Being kind and going the extra mile to engage in an act of service, to say something encouraging, or to make time to listen is one of the most important things I can do with my time, and it can trump other commitments.	Parent	• I demonstrate kindness to my parent by making sure that I help with tasks that are getting challenging for them as they get older, being patient when they need help, and giving my full attention to them. • My parent demonstrates kindness to me by listening to me and giving me perspective and wisdom when I need it.

Linking your values, beliefs, and boundaries to a specific person and the reciprocity between you can be an important exercise to explore the overall health and function of your closest relationships. An important piece of this puzzle is the demonstration of these values: are others demonstrating them to you and are you demonstrating them to others? We sometimes take our closest relationships for granted, which means that we slack off about giving the best version of ourselves to the people we're closest to. When this happens, we're not as kind as we could be, or we become harsh in our feedback or conversations, which may mean that our honest messages are not heard. Questions that we must ask ourselves include: What does it look like when my intimate relationships are working well? What does it look like when they're not working well? When you think about the answers to these questions, consider how you feel, think, and act when your intimate relationships are working well and when they feel "off."

INNER CIRCLE EXERCISE

It's your turn. Consider the values that you hold about your intimate relationships and the people with whom you share those relationships. Use table 6.2 to write your thoughts.

Table 6.2. Inner Circle Reflection Exercise

Value	Belief	Boundary	Person	Demonstration

REFLECTION QUESTIONS

When answering the questions below, consider how you react to the people closest to you and how they may be reacting to you.

- What does it look like when my intimate relationships are working well?
- What does it look like when they're not working well?

KEYSTONES OF INTIMATE RELATIONSHIPS

When we are trying to understand our closest relationships, sometimes it's important to take a step back to give ourselves some perspective on the key components that support them. My short list of the most important components for our closest relationships includes honesty, variety, evolution, and safety to be vulnerable. Let's start with two that I believe are closely linked, which are variety and honesty. In my own life, I have found that it is unrealistic for me to expect that one specific relationship will meet all my emotional needs. I know that some people have found that a single relationship or partner meets most of their needs. Anecdotally, I haven't seen this to be the case very often. Some argue that sharing your deepest self with people other than your romantic partner may be dangerous to your relationship. Often people think about emotional affairs when these issues come up. An emotional affair is a deeply emotional relationship with someone other than your romantic partner. These relationships can sometimes lead to sexual relationships. The major sign that signals an emotional affair is secrecy. Hiding a relationship, your texts, or conversations with another person or lying altogether to your partner about your other relationships indicates a bigger relationship problem. If you find that secrecy and subterfuge are major parts of your most important relationships, it could mean that those relationships are not healthy.

So what does it mean to have healthy, intimate relationships? Thinking back to where we started, *honesty* is the most important keystone in our closest relationships, and part of honesty is asserting boundaries and communicating rules and limits of the relationship. Consider the role that honesty plays in your current intimate relationships; some of our roles include mother, partner, daughter, sister, friend, aunt. We sometimes negotiate these important relationships without much thought because they are so ingrained in our daily lives. They deserve more intentionality because they are some of the richest and most meaningful connections in our lives. Some of us are afraid of honesty because we may have had experiences where it feels aggressive or confrontational. However, honesty means being true to how you're feeling, thinking, and behaving and sharing your truth with the people who are closest to you in the healthiest way possible. Conveying your honesty will not always go perfectly or be easy, and yet it is one of the pieces of communication that can strengthen your relationships.

Another keystone is acknowledging the rich *variety* of intimate relationships that we can have in life. In my life, this shift has helped me to broaden my perspective regarding how many indispensable people who represent different types of love that I have in my inner circle. Harkening back to the list of love types, how many are represented in your life? I'm hopeful that you'll recognize two or more, and you find that these relationships bring richness to your life experience. What is beautiful about having a variety of close relationships is the opportunity to include people in your life who have known you at different ages and stages. These close relationships also can reflect how you have grown and evolved over time.

Evolution, knowing that all of us have the potential to change as we move through our lives, is another keystone to intimate relationships. One of the most important aspects of a lasting intimate relationship is understanding that change is inevitable. If you have known people who were resistant to changes you've gone through, wanted you to stay exactly the same, it may have felt constricting. In our close relationships, we hope to grow and change together. We try to accept that although these evolutions may feel difficult or threatening, it is important to honor the person's journey. An example that comes to mind is when you blaze a new path that may not be one that is familiar to the people you love. Imagine you decide to change your career in midlife, maybe taking a lower-paying job so that you can gain entrance into a new field. Your people may show some concern about this change for a variety of reasons, maybe even by not supporting your decision, sometimes very vocally. I think of my sister who was worried about a life decision that I made. She showed her care by expressing her concern that I would regret my choice. She showed her love through reminding me about her concerns, and it was up to me to interpret her words not as an attack, but the way she shows she cares for me.

One of the bravest things that you can do in this life is to try something new and evolve. Just like a hermit crab is at its most vulnerable when it leaves its old shell to find a bigger one, you are vulnerable every time you dare to change. You want your inner circle to be the people who surround you and emotionally protect you as you find your new shell. This can be a hard thing for the people who care about you, because sometimes protecting you means voicing concerns that you're on a path that may not be healthy or have long-term benefit to you. People who want the best for you often want to protect you from hardships, which is an inherent part of change. Those who are close to you learn the balance between expressing care, supporting while providing feedback when you get offtrack, and helping and celebrating as you move through your life path and evolve into the person whom you are working to become. This is a balance that you must learn as you reciprocate your love and care to others.

Finally, the *safety to be vulnerable* is one of the last keystones that makes up my short list of important characteristics in intimate relationships. When you feel safe with another person, you feel protected from harm, danger, and judgment. This means that you can be vulnerable and share the deepest parts of your soul. An example of this for me is when I am moved to tears. I don't cry often, but when I do cry, it's typically in front of people I feel safe with. Those who see my tears tend to be my most intimate family and friends. These people are also the recipients of my first phone calls and texts when something good happens. Using the shell metaphor above, these are the people who have seen me without my protective shell. Thinking of these intimate relationship keystones, consider the following:

- Who are the people who see your deepest vulnerabilities? How do you know that they are safe and have earned the privilege of access to your inner world?
- Are you sharing your most vulnerable self, or have you shied away from sharing yourself with others?
- What part do these relationship keystones play in your intimate relationships?

Answers to these questions are helpful when evaluating the strength of your closest relationships.

WHEN LOVE BECOMES TOXIC

Toxicity in relationships can be like the frog in boiling water analogy: a frog placed in cool water that's slowly heated won't notice when the water is boiling, an environment the frog won't survive. Toxic elements in a relationship can include jealousy, dishonesty, isolation, blaming, ongoing conflict, gaslighting, and coercion. Intimate relationships can contain any of these elements to some degree, and they can recover from them if all parties are aware and want to work to detoxify the situation. It can take a great deal of work and commitment to change patterns in a relationship, and sliding back into old patterns is easy. Keep in mind that love that becomes toxic is harmful and isn't loving. You can love someone who is toxic and be in an intimate relationship with them, but there will be emotional consequences. Let's explore how we can find ourselves in this situation.

Our earliest relationships tend to be with our parents or caregivers and can influence how we engage in intimate relationships for the rest of our lives. The idea makes sense because being cared for as a young child is one of the most vulnerable and intimate experiences of our lives. How we experience these first relationships is explained through theories of attachment and attachment styles. Attachment theory is the study of the relationships between people and is based on the notion that young children's experiences with their caregivers can form the basis for their ability to build relationships throughout their lives. John Bowlby is the researcher most associated with attachment theory, and he pioneered the idea along with operational definitions of the different attachment styles for infants (Scharfe, Pitman, & Cole, 2017). Bowlby's research is still relevant today, and researchers continue to use his initial work to build upon current theories and interventions. Although Bowlby's work focused on young children, there are some adaptations of attachment language for adults that are useful when thinking about relationship styles.

For adults, these attachment styles are defined as follows: (1) *secure*: individuals who can be emotionally close to others and who feel comfortable that they can depend on others and have others depend on them; (2) *fearful*: individuals who are somewhat uncomfortable being close to others, who may have difficulty trusting or being too dependent on others, who may be concerned about being hurt by others; (3) *preoccupied*: individuals who want to be emotionally close to others but find that others are not as willing to be emotionally close to them, who may worry that they are not as valued as they value others; (4) *dismissing*: individuals who are comfortable not having close relationships, who prefer to feel independent and self-sufficient without others depending on them (Feeney & Noller, 1996; Scharfe, Pitman, & Cole, 2017).

Using attachment as a jumping-off point, let's start with traits of toxic parenting, which refers to an unhealthy parenting style that shows disregard for children's needs and autonomy, unrealistic expectations for children to perform certain tasks or achieve, lack of empathy for children's experiences, dismissal of children's lived experiences, high levels of parental control over children's lives and activities, and high levels of criticism of children's efforts (Harahap & Daulay, 2023). Imagine a girl in your fourth-grade class, let's call her Jillian, who may have been unsure that her voice or opinions mattered. She had a high need to achieve and was extremely anxious if she didn't, to the point of crying or becoming very upset and withdrawn if she failed. She may have felt overly responsible for other people's feelings, consistently apologizing if she thought she had upset someone. She also may not have participated in extracurricular events because her parents wouldn't allow it or restricted her activities because they took away from family time. In more extreme instances, she may have shown signs of neglect, physical abuse, or sexual abuse.

As she grows up, Jillian may find herself gravitating toward toxic friendships. We seek out friendships to foster a sense of belonging and to feel less isolated and lonely in the world. Humans are not built to be in isolation; we're naturally social creatures, and friendships are one of the ways that we fulfill this need. Jillian may find that there are imbalances within her friendships; perhaps she gives more emotional support than her friends do. She also may find that her "friends" will use humiliation tactics or rejection to get her to do what they want. Even though her friendships cause her emotional distress, she may remain in them because she wants to belong to a group. Her past experiences with her family may have taught her that this is how relationships work and that her role in relationships is to be overaccommodating, to walk on eggshells, and to believe (incorrectly) that she should have low self-esteem because she is somehow not as good as her friends are.

At some point, Jillian may start dating and find a romantic partner that she stays with long term. Let's think about how Jillian's beliefs about herself and others may set her up to find someone who may not treat her well. She may have grown accustomed to putting her own needs last; she may have low self-esteem due to being told by those close to her that she falls short in her achievements, looks, and so on; she may have a very limited circle of people who show interest in her unless they want something from her; she also may be emotionally fragile and therefore seen as weak. Honestly, this list makes me worried for Jillian and other women I've met who are like her. Her experiences may lead her to find a romantic partner who is emotionally abusive and whose behavior may escalate into physical, sexual, or other types of abuse.

Although Jillian's story may not sound familiar to you, some of my readers may feel emotional because they recognize either parts or all of Jillian's story in their own or someone they love. Take a breath and honor that insight; it is a powerful one. Toxicity in relationships occurs along a spectrum, and we all can have some toxic traits or occurrences in our relationships. For example, a fight that escalates and results in two people not speaking for a period can be an indicator of toxicity. Relationship disengagement, in which individuals stop making an effort to connect and allow the relationship to wither can be considered toxic. The point is that no relationship is perfect and there are times when all of us are susceptible to using toxic methods to have our voices heard within an intimate relationship. The questions to ask yourself are: Are you experiencing toxicity in your relationships often? If there are toxic traits in some of your relationships, how do they impact you? Despite your identified levels of relationship toxicity, do you believe that you have healthy relationships?

Many of the types of love that you can experience have the potential to become toxic given the opportunity and right conditions. We must be vigilant about our own behavior and acknowledge when we observe toxic behavior in our relationships with other people. We can only control ourselves; we can't control the people we're in relationships with.

Rather, we must know the warning signs and acknowledge that if we're in a toxic relationship, there are serious consequences to our mental health. I have worked with women who remain in many types of toxic relationships: with their parents, friends, religious communities, and romantic partners. They believe that they cannot leave these relationships. For some of us, that is true. We remain in certain toxic relationships because it is familiar, comfortable, or the thought of not having a relationship with the person is more painful than having a challenging one.

One of the best analogies I ever heard about living in a toxic relationship came from a woman who discussed how she negotiated her relationship with her narcissistic mother. This woman, whom I'll call Charity (age forty-two), shared that her mother consistently demanded her attention and help, was critical of the help that was offered her, and became enraged if Charity found different or better solutions for her mother's issues. Charity described her love for her mother and acknowledged that she knew that her mother's ability to love her was limited. Charity wanted to have a relationship with her because her mother was one of her few living biological relatives. What Charity described as her boundary with this toxic loved one was a "half-wall." The image that comes to me is almost like the circular brick enclosure around the opening of a well, with Charity standing inside the brick circle. In her safe circle, Charity could see her mother and interact with her if she wanted or needed to, but the boundary prevented her mother from getting too close to her.

Owning Your Own Toxicity

I started this book with a story about my midlife crisis and how I thought I didn't want to be married anymore. Spoiler alert: I'm still married. Second spoiler alert: my husband is the hero of this story. One of my intimate relationships, my romantic relationship, became toxic mostly because I didn't tend to it. Don't get me wrong; there are two people in our relationship, and he bears his share of responsibility. And I was the one who became distant and disengaged. I was the one who was jealous of his free time because I chose to be a workaholic (still in recovery). I was the one who blamed him when things weren't done to my standards (recovering perfectionist also). I was the one who didn't want to compromise on certain decisions (raised without my significantly older siblings in the home and in essence the only child—what is compromise anyway?).

So what happened? In a very dramatic, solo, and silent ashram experience, I realized that the roots of many of the problems in my romantic relationship were me. If I wanted to stay in the relationship, I was going to have to get vulnerable with myself and my partner to figure out a way to change and bring a *much better* version of myself to our relationship. The first thing it took was removing myself from the situation temporarily to get some perspective and clarity. Then I needed to communicate to my partner that perhaps my declaration about not wanting to be married anymore was a bit hasty. It also took asking for help in the form of couples counseling and individual counseling to see what toxic behaviors I engaged in as an individual and what toxic behaviors and traits we engaged in as a couple that hurt our relationship. This work began our progress toward resuscitating our relationship and making it healthier and stronger.

Was it easy? No. Was it fun? No, I can think of far better ways to spend date night than in a therapist's office. And I'm a therapist. But it was worth it. This is my person. He is one of the select people who is in my inner circle, who knows my secrets, and who loves me still. A few weeks after my father died it was my birthday. My partner gave me a gift that I thought was a fancy box of chocolates. Imagine my surprise when I opened the box and it held a beautiful necklace with a heart pendant. The first thought that popped into my head was, "I'm going to be okay. Despite how sad and bruised I feel, here is a person who shows up for me and loves and cares for me." Did I need a necklace to show me that? No, what I needed was to get out of my own way and see the core beauty of this relationship we've built over the last twenty-plus years.

When you're reflecting on your relationships, some are worth saving and can be saved because the people in them are willing to put in the work to create change. There are some relationships, like Charity's, that you keep because the pain of losing them is greater than the pain of keeping them. There are some relationships that you leave or let go because remaining in them is more harmful than not. Not all relationships are meant to last; there are healthy and functional relationships that fade away because they were not meant to be lifelong. Short-term relationships can be just as important in the arc of your story and are no less valuable. If you discover that a relationship is toxic or that you are toxic in a relationship and you need to exit, doing so is okay. It might be hard and painful, but you aren't required to stay in relationships if they no longer work and you've done what you can to make them healthy. Even if you promised your sixth-grade best friend you'd be BFFs, sometimes it still doesn't work out.

Keep in mind that toxicity can include your relationship with yourself because all of us are prone to egocentrism in our lives, where the focus is all on ourselves. This can emerge because of a crisis or because we're in stressful situations. But when we move into narcissism, where there is no room for others' interests or we think about other people's experiences solely through the lens of how it affects us personally, that is problematic. You may start to notice that your closest friends or family distance themselves from you. This can be a clue that you are becoming toxic to them, and it is time to engage in some personal reflection.

BRING YOUR BEST SELF TO THE INNER CIRCLE

We've discussed the keystones of intimate relationships: honesty, variety, evolution, and the safety to be vulnerable. These are the conditions of the relationship, and the relationship is only as functional as the people who are in it. What I mean by this is that to have the healthiest intimate relationships you can, you must show up as the healthiest version of yourself that you can. If you aren't healthy, then it's up to you to take responsibility for working toward becoming healthier. Remember me saying (and taking responsibility for) that it was (largely) me who created a toxic relationship with my partner? What makes that important is that I am holding myself accountable for my actions in my relationship. How do you need to hold yourself accountable? If you are unhealthy in your relationships, other people already know—it's not a secret. However, there is power in taking responsibility for issues you've created and taking real steps to make amends and change as needed.

What does it mean to take responsibility? For some it means saying it out loud; for others, it means writing a letter. Taking responsibility means admitting that you didn't bring the best of yourself to your most important relationships. When you take responsibility, you are empowered to evolve into a more functional and healthier person in your relationship with the people you care about the most. Taking responsibility means that you value your relationships and will work to show those you care for that they are important to you.

What does it take to maintain your healthy relationships or to work toward greater health? The first thing is taking care of your shit. That can mean reflecting on what is and isn't working and going to individual or couples/family counseling (I've counseled friend groups who were engaged in toxic patterns; don't let the name "couple" or "family" lead you to believe that you can't bring friends and chosen family to therapy). It might mean saying yes to trying something new or saying no to extricate yourself from activities that aren't healthy; maybe you're doing it through reading this or other books. Ultimately, being in committed, intimate relationships with the people in your inner circle means committing to bring your best self to the relationships. This doesn't mean all the time—we are not our best selves all the time—but we need to show up often as this healthy version.

WHAT DOES IT FEEL LIKE WHEN IT'S WORKING WELL?

I've just returned from my annual girl's weekend trip. We've all known each other for more than twenty years and started having an annual get-together every year to connect now that our lives are busy and scattered. Together we've celebrated weddings, babies, and new jobs; we've buried parents, supported each other through family troubles, and stayed close during health crises. I am beyond grateful to have found these strong and smart women whom I trust implicitly. I was struck this last visit by how we've entered a "grateful" era, meaning we are much more open and vocal about how grateful we are that we have these long-lasting friendships. I think it is because we know how special it can be for people to have healthy, long-term relationships that have survived and thrived over many years and changes. I know our relationships work well because we share some of our deepest thoughts and struggles; we respect each other's boundaries; and we know that we want the very best for each other and support each other through all the changes that we've been through as individuals.

When our intimate relationships are working well, it feels like magic, like you are united by love and purpose, that there are no limits to what you can do. There is a certainty to feeling loved and secure; there is something beautiful about being able to create a sense of love for the people closest to you so that they can share this wonderful feeling. To create the optimal situation for these feelings, we must start with ourselves. When we love ourselves, when we have the surety of whom we are in relationships, then we can offer the best version of ourselves to those we care about most deeply.

There is a moment in February 2021 that I remember so vividly. I'm sitting on my couch and crying. I had been hospitalized a few months earlier and was still recovering, my father had died in January, my family felt chaotic, and the world felt chaotic because we were in a pandemic. My partner came into the living room and sat down with me. He didn't touch me or try to hug me, he sat observing me cry. He then said, "You've been through so much, and it's okay to cry. I'm going to sit with you while you do." That moment is better than any love note he ever wrote me. My partner knew me so well, and he knew what I needed in that moment: those tears were something that only I could experience, but I didn't want to be alone with my feelings. I was required to evolve a lot over ten weeks, and this man was there to help me feel safe and was honest in expressing to me that he wasn't always sure he was helping me in the "right" way but that he would be there to support me. Although I had many people in my life who supported me at that time, he was certainly the person who supported me the most.

"HOW HEALTHY IS YOUR POND?" EXERCISE

Just like our frog in boiling water, your inner circle is like a pond whose health depends on the level of toxicity in the water. The more toxic traits in your pond, the more polluted the water. The more polluted the water, the worse you feel. For this exercise, consider how many toxic and healthy traits exist in your most important relationships and draw a hash mark for each category. For a pond to be healthy, the healthy traits should outweigh the toxic ones. Table 6.3 shows an example.

Table 6.3. Sample Evaluating Traits in Relationships Exercise

Relationship	Toxic Traits	Healthy Traits
Sibling	III	I

Next, if you have more toxic than healthy traits, put a snake in the pond (figure 6.2).

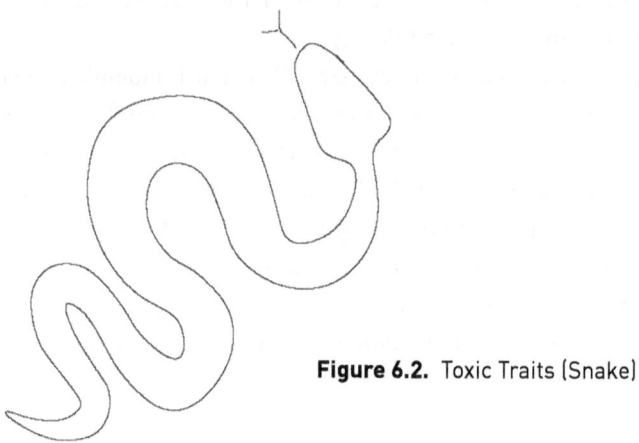

Figure 6.2. Toxic Traits (Snake)

If you have more healthy than toxic traits in the pond, put a fish in the pond (figure 6.3).

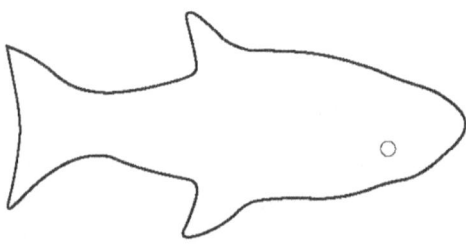

Figure 6.3. Healthy Traits (Fish)

For the example below, figure 6.4 shows a snake in the pond.

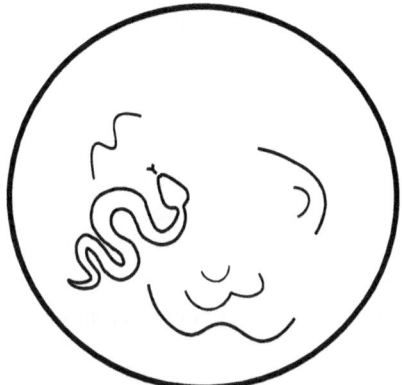

Figure 6.4. A Relationship "Pond" with a Toxic Trait (Snake in the Pond)

Using table 6.4, reflect on your intimate relationships and the traits therein. Using figure 6.5, you can create your pond so that you have a visual representation of its health.

Table 6.4. Evaluating Traits in Intimate Relationships Exercise

Relationship	Toxic Traits	Healthy Traits

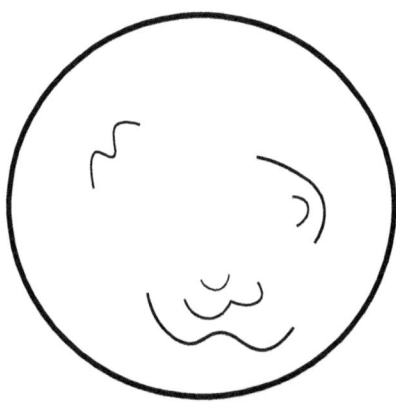

Figure 6.5. Pond Exercise

REFLECTION QUESTIONS

Finally, consider these closing questions as you reflect on your most important and intimate relationships:

- Which relationships are you most proud of?
- Do you have more snakes or fish in your pond?
- Do you see any toxic traits that are patterns in your relationships?
- What can you do to "detoxify" your pond?
- What steps can you take to resuscitate a toxic relationship—or to determine whether to let it go?
- What boundaries do you need to establish in your intimate relationships?

Having healthy relationships begins with those closest to us, but many of the same principles and practices (especially setting boundaries) apply—and in some cases are even more necessary—to how we show up in public and interact as part of a community. In the next chapter, we look at our social connections—the circle just beyond our inner one—and how these can impact our journey, and how we may need to refine this circle for this stage of life.

CHAPTER SEVEN

SOCIAL HEALTH

There I was, sitting in session with a client who was scrolling through her socials feed to show me something that she considered to be outrageous that one of her friends had posted.

My client: You're not going to believe what she said. And once you see the post, I want to show you the text chain we had going after this incident. It just went on and on. Finally, I stopped responding and we haven't communicated since.

Me: So you want to connect more with your friend and work through this conflict, but you are only interacting through social media and texting?

My client: Yes, our lives are busy and even though we're in the same town, we really don't get together all that often. We keep in touch through feeds. I hate conflict, so I think that communicating through text is easier and helps me stay calmer.

Me: Hmm . . . I know we've talked about how you've been lonely and needing to connect with others and how you want to work on your communication skills. I'm wondering if there may be some opportunities for growing those skills here?

My client: Maybe, but can you just look at the posts and tell me what you think?

Lots of clients come to my office with big problems, and one of the biggest problems they face is how to stay socially connected. The struggle to connect isn't unique to any gender or age group. In 2023 the World Health Organization declared loneliness a global public health concern and the US surgeon general declared loneliness a public health crisis (Christensen, 2023; Jaffe, 2023). People are working hard to connect with one another, particularly in the face of loneliness. Loneliness coupled with the world pandemic contributed greatly to a change in the way we experience our social ties. Many have used technology and social media to combat loneliness and expand their social networks, but these mechanisms can be a double-edged sword. Technology can be a great way to stay abreast of what is going on with loved ones near and far, but prolonged and intensive use of social media can increase feelings of loneliness and depression.

When I talk about your social circle, I'm referring to folks who are outside of your intimate relationships, such as coworkers, less intimate friends and family, acquaintances, and others you see as connected to you. Our social circle can consist of real-life and online connections, with some relationships occurring in both the real and virtual worlds. Just like my client, we often try to use social media as an outlet to stay connected and stave off boredom and loneliness. Have you ever had the experience of being upset because one of your favorite people to follow (be it a person in your social circle or an influencer you follow) hasn't posted on socials recently? No one in the virtual world owes you anything, and yet you may feel upset because they're not posting and "staying in touch." These parasocial relationships are one-sided and may not be as emotionally fulfilling to us in the long term, and yet we engage in them. I think this is such an interesting phenomenon of which I am a victim as well. I want to be connected beyond my inner circle, and one of the ways that I fill the void is to connect on a virtual platform as well as in real life (IRL). Furthermore, like the client I mentioned earlier, many folks are either unable or less willing to connect with others through face-to-face or phone interaction. By not flexing our in-person socialization muscles, we are losing the ability to create and maintain meaningful connections, which are cornerstones of our overall health and happiness.

Our goal in this chapter is to determine the right balance between virtual and real-life interactions so that you can maintain a healthy social life and figure out how to be real in an unreal world. Social relationships are one or two levels removed from your inner circle and can be considered your outward or public life. Our social lives include people we interact with every day, but we usually do this without analyzing how they impact us—in this chapter, we are going to analyze them. We're also going to look at sticky situations, such as conflict, and how to negotiate it in a healthy way that honors differences and maintains your values. With respect to our social health, we're lucky we're in the middle. We didn't grow up with social media and we were socialized in our early lives in ways that are very similar to our parents. This is a strength because we have enjoyed both worlds and can switch between virtual interaction and real-life interaction and have skills in both.

WHO IS IN YOUR SOCIAL NETWORK?

In the last chapter, we did a deep dive into your inner circle. One insight you may have had is that folks who were previously in your inner circle may have moved into one of the outer circles. This can be particularly true in friendships that have evolved or that you've outgrown, relationships that are strained by distance or lack of time and commitment. Your outer circles can include friends, family members, coworkers, and community members who are less privy to your intimate life. As in the previous chapter, use figure 7.1 to write the names of people who are in your second and third outer social circles.

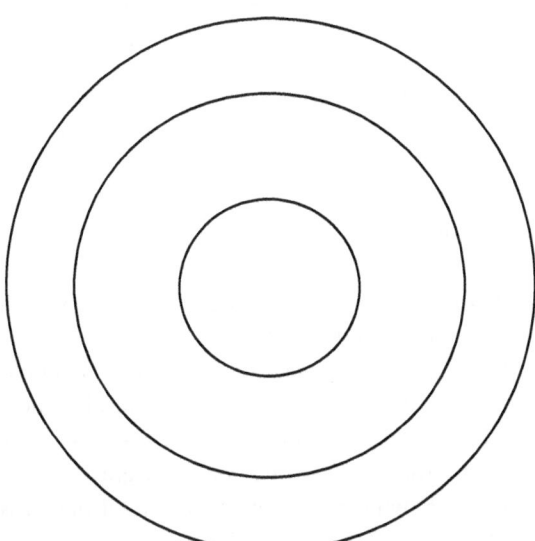

Figure 7.1. Your Outer Social Circles

As you write the names of these individuals, consider who is in your social network by choice and who is there due to circumstances. This is an important distinction that speaks to the level of control you have in your social network. Ideally, most of the folks in your social network are connected to you by choice; however, most of us live in the reality that there are some people in our lives whom we would not choose. They can include friends of friends, coworkers or bosses, or members of organizations or interest groups you belong to.

Thinking back to your values regarding relationships, you may find that you can pull similar values from our last chapter or that you want to include new values that you didn't include in the last chapter. I encourage you to make this exercise a mix of people who are in your social circle by choice and those who are not, those who are easy to be around and those who are not. Using such a mix is helpful in solidifying your image of yourself in your social life. See an example of this exercise in table 7.1 and use table 7.2 to complete your reflection. Use additional paper as needed if you want to complete a more extensive inventory of your social relationships.

REFLECTION QUESTIONS

As you review your inventory, there are several questions you may wish to consider concerning your social relationships. These can include:

- Who are you in your public life? We all engage in different roles or may wear "masks" for different facets of our lives. Is the person you are in your public life congruent with your values? Think about how this may or may not be true for you.
- How do you manage your energy? Your social relationships can take as much or as little energy as you wish to put in. How are you managing this energy in a way that is healthy for you and allows you to engage in all the areas of your life you wish to live?
- How do you measure your social health? What is "enough" or "not enough" in terms of social relationships? We all function along a spectrum with some folks needing more or less from their social relationships than others: Where do you fall right now? Is that satisfying for you? If so, what makes it satisfying? If not, what makes it unsatisfying?

Table 7.1. Sample Reflection on Social Relationships

Value	Belief	Person	Boundary	Limits of the Relationship
Honesty	Telling the truth is part of showing trust	Co-worker	Sharing honest feedback is important. Since I don't trust this person, I will share limited information with them: enough interaction to keep work running smoothly, but nothing personal or intimate so that I can feel safe. This includes limited real-life interactions and blocking them on personal social media accounts and other virtual platforms.	This relationship is toxic due to a work conflict. There is limited mutual trust in the relationship, and the damage is currently not repairable.
Kindness	Showing kindness to important people in my life is one of the ways I show love and care.	Friend	Being kind and going the extra mile to engage in an act of service, to say something encouraging, or to make time to listen is one of the most important things I can do with my time, and it can trump other commitments.	This is a healthy relationship but is limited by our mutual outside and family commitments. I will make space for our get-togethers and commit to our monthly meetings while maintaining flexibility and grace for each of us as we manage the seasons of our lives.

Table 7.2. Reflection on Social Relationships

Value	Belief	Person	Boundary	Limits of the Relationship

OUR SOCIAL LIVES MAY CHANGE DURING MIDLIFE

Our midyears can be a busy time in our lives, with family, work, and other obligations. The hope is that, as we mature and become more comfortable in our skin, we may be less wrapped up in how other people think about us. I believe this is a work in progress; I admire folks who blithely go through life without caring about what others think. I am an internal processor, so while it may seem as if I don't care, because I may not outwardly show it or talk about it, I care deeply about how other people perceive me and tend to internalize a lot of false beliefs because of this trait. My work on my social anxiety has taken me a lifetime, and I am still working on it. I'm not done dispelling internalized beliefs that I imprint from others. So if you fall into this category, you have lots of company. However, there are some insights that I think we all have at this stage of our lives that can free us from worrying about what others may think.

The first insight is that our time is finite, and we know that now more than ever. We have also tried a lot of things and have started to figure out and home in on what gives us the most fulfillment. We have reached a point when we've experienced enough life that we can make better decisions about which social interactions give us the most payoff, engaging in those rather than other activities that we feel obligated to do. For example, I have spent the last few years as a member of a professional women's sorority. I seldom attend regular meetings, and during more recent meetings, I've noticed that I don't connect with the members in the same way that I have in the past. As I reflected on this group, I realized that I was rejoining more out of habit and a sense of obligation rather than true desire. My actions reflected this, even when I was available to attend meetings, I consistently declined. Balancing this commitment with my others, I realized that I was doing something that I didn't enjoy, spending money on dues for limited return, and feeling internalized pressure that I was somehow "failing," when in fact I had simply moved past wanting to be part of this organization. So I quit the group. Don't get me wrong, these thoughts had circled my head for a while before I finally quit. And when I did leave this group, it felt great, like I was finally being true to myself. It also opened my headspace and calendar to engage in social activities that better aligned with who I am now.

Another way that our social spheres tend to change is through life events that shrink our circles. Midlife can bring with it changes in partnership status, like divorce. We also may change jobs, relocate to a new place, begin working from home without officemates, develop health issues, and care for children, parents, or others who need our nurturance and time. Studies have shown that compared to their younger and older counterparts, midlife women report more stressors due to external factors (such as caregiving) as well as their changing health status (Thomas, Mitchell, Woods, 2018). Juggling co-occurring stressors can take a lot of time and attention, which doesn't leave a lot of energy for social relationships. This is a challenge because we know that social connections can keep people healthy and grounded, yet stressors can often lead women toward anxiety and depression, a symptom of which can be social withdrawal.

Another set of issues that can occur in midlife is that we may have less energy and focus, and our energy is spread more thinly. This certainly can be due to the stressors mentioned, but it also can be brought about by biological changes that we may experience during this time, such as menopause. What I see many women attempting to do when faced with this obstacle is to "push through" and function on autopilot just to keep things moving. This may be functional in the short term but can cause long-term consequences. Often when we are on autopilot, we ignore what our emotions or physical body is trying to tell us. Functioning on autopilot can result in not being fully present for the people we socialize with or in diminished enjoyment when engaging with people and activities that we previously enjoyed.

When we ignore the messages our emotions and body are trying to send us, we disrupt the naturally occurring internal mechanisms that help us to maintain balance. Having less focus and then choosing to not focus and check in on ourselves can result in us not engaging in the healthiest and most fulfilling social lives that we could have. These are the forces that are within us; let's also consider outside forces that impact our social lives.

OUR SOCIAL LIVES HAVE CHANGED AS A SOCIETY

As I mentioned, I allowed my membership to lapse in one of my community organizations. Although I've maintained other commitments, I've become much more selective about how I spend my time. I bet you have too. A great deal of information shows that membership organizations, church involvement, social groups, and so forth lack the robust attendance and membership retention rates that they had in the past

(Tsipursky, 2023). The lessening of face-to-face interaction has been a slow trend that gained momentum during the pandemic when social distancing became the norm.

Coupled with this trend is an uptick in the number of folks who are working from home (WFH). WFH arrangements can give us more flexibility but also make it challenging to maintain social connections with others in our work community (Haan, 2023). Something that can ease this burden is the use of digital formats to stay connected, through social media platforms, text messages, online meeting platforms, virtual gaming, and so on. Additionally, our work lives continue to take a great deal of our time, with more people reporting that they work more than forty hours per week and "check in" to the office even during their nonworking hours. As a result, more of our social life involves the people with whom we work, which isn't a bad thing, although it may blur the lines between work and leisure life in a way that limits rejuvenation away from work.

Perhaps you've also noticed that as we've shifted to more virtual platforms for connection, our social lives have been both enhanced and muddied by famous stars and influencers with ulterior motives for sharing their experiences to gain and maintain profit and celebrity. Don't get me wrong, I think it is great fun to see Viola Davis's reposts of funny memes and celebrity status updates, but if I'm not careful, I'm following lots of folks who aren't personal friends, which in the short term can be fun, but in the long term isn't really meaningful social connection.

I believe that virtual social connection can be as vital to our lives as real-life interactions; however, we must be very mindful of its limitations as well. Let me explain by taking a step back and talking about the limbic system. Our limbic system is made up of complex brain structures that are responsible for emotions, motivation, memory, and behavior regulation. The cool part about this is that when we are engaged with others in intimate or social relationships, our limbic system is affected, which is called limbic resonance. Think about meeting a friend and attuning to each other's emotional output during a conversation. For example, I had breakfast with a friend and colleague who shared some hard stories about her life, and as we moved through the conversation, we attuned to one another's needs, offering emotional support and troubleshooting some challenging issues.

These real-life interactions promote limbic resonance, in which our limbic systems sync with one another; this mutual influence is called limbic regulation. How our limbic system interacts with the limbic systems of others can profoundly influence our emotional well-being and personality development (Lewis, Amini, & Lannon, 2001). When individuals' brains are attuned to each other, our feelings of connectedness, emotional understanding, and empathy increase. Here's the thing: the most profound way to experience limbic resonance is through real-life interactions, not online interactions. A quote from work by my colleague Dr. Amanda Giordano (2021) sums it up here:

> It is important to note that although social media users may be striving for belonging, the virtual realm may not be an effective means of meeting that need. Indeed, Savci and Aysan (2017) found that social media addiction was associated with decreased social connectedness among adolescents. Moreover, in their discussion of limbic resonance (i.e., the experience in which the neuronal patterns of two human beings become synchronized when they are attuned to one another), Lewis, Amini, and Lannon (2001) reported that the internet is a poor substitute for in-person, face-to-face connections. Thus, evidence suggests that online, virtual connections may not be as fulfilling as offline relationships.

So what does this mean for us as we navigate an increasingly online world? We can get social fulfillment through our virtual platforms, but our brains do not experience the same type of connection that they receive in real-life relationships and interactions. Additionally, these online connections may not yield the same self-regulation benefits that real-life relationships do. This is, again, where being in midlife is a superpower. We grew up before the ubiquity of internet connection, so we had to develop the skills necessary to connect with others IRL. We've reaped the benefits of these connections, and we (hopefully) have achieved some long-lasting social connections that satisfy us. We also are able to navigate the virtual world, having experienced its advent and participating in its growth and evolution.

The good thing is that the balance of abilities allows us to maintain our healthy real-life social relationships, with the skills that we need to nurture them. Our online relationships can increase our social network and expand our connections, but also enable us to influence others, maintain relationships with people who are "like" us, and gather followers from far beyond our geographical sphere of influence. Some of us pursue our online social lives with ulterior motives, to expand our sphere of influence, to exchange ideas that can help us grow in some way, and to pursue greater levels of social success through likes and followers. These motivations can help us grow our social circles, but they aren't necessarily as satisfying or fulfilling nor do they feel as good as real-life relationships that allow for connection and limbic resonance.

I think we're all trying to figure out the social norms in this new community we've created, a liminal space that includes both real-life and virtual interactions. Though I believe we are trying our best to determine how we fit into this new world, there is a real struggle among us to figure out how to proceed. Women are naturally relational, so I can see how we see the virtual world as a tool to help us expand how we connect with others. But like my client at the beginning of the chapter, some miscommunications can happen in this space, which can have ramifications on how we interact with each other both in person and virtually. And, as a counselor, I've seen a growing trend in which individuals are readily willing to "quit" their friendships over minor conflict. Let me be clear: it is completely healthy to leave a relationship that is not healthy. However, I am referring to situations in which individuals simply stop interacting and avoid each other rather than attempting to resolve a conflict. Or worse, they begin to attack each other in the virtual world rather than resolve issues that create conflict. Have you seen this level of animosity in your social networks?

Part of the reason that we see this discord is that our online lives give us easy accessibility to our social networks, relative anonymity to explore new social networks, and limited accountability for engaging in bad behavior toward others. These three A's, along with a lack of autonomy in controlling our virtual social lives, have concerned scholars since the online world became a social force (Branscomb, 1995). In the next section, we take a deeper dive into these three A's and their implications for our lives. But first, let's take some time to discuss *harmonious disagreement*, a concept that can help us find common ground with others who don't share our values. Spoiler alert: the longer you know someone, the more you will realize that you don't share every single value in common.

HARMONIOUS DISAGREEMENT

One of the things that I believe we all struggle with is managing relationships with people when we don't share the same values. The reality is that each of us values different things—and along a spectrum—so what I value and how much I value it is very different from what and how you value the same concept. One example might be loyalty. I value being loyal to my commitments, which can include things like brands. I have been using the same brand of soap since I was a child, and I'm deeply attached to it. It's not as popular anymore, so it's harder to find. Also, if I researched it, it's probably not as good for my skin as other types of soap. But I keep coming back to it, even when I branch out and try other things. There are several reasons for this, likely due to familiarity, comfort, and so forth. But ultimately, I think that my value of loyalty brings me back to this bar of soap.

Contrast that with someone who also values loyalty but to a lesser degree (particularly as it relates to something as inane as soap). This might be a person who tries a particular brand of soap and enjoys it, but staying loyal to a commitment for them might mean comparing other types of soap so that they know that what they are staying loyal to is really the best for them. It doesn't make them disloyal; it means that they are a bit more flexible in how they value loyalty. Neither tactic is wrong; it's simply a different style of being. Taking this a step further, imagine if this other person and I got into an argument about the value of loyalty, me with my staunch soap beliefs and her with her more flexible ones. We might fight about soap, but really what we're arguing about is our value of loyalty, how we each interpret the merits of the value, and how we embody the value in our lives. Each of our interpretations is our own—it is correct for us—but our interpretations may not align with each other. If we are stuck in our interpretation of how loyalty "should" be demonstrated and believe we are "right," then we may get into an even more heated discourse about the "right" way to be loyal. Neither of us will win the argument by trying to sway the other to our side because what works for one of us doesn't work for both of us.

You can imagine where I'm going with this. We live in a culture in which people want to be "right" and believe that what they value should be the commonly held values for all. Sometimes that works and sometimes it doesn't. There are some values I think we can all mutually agree on, like people have the right to feel safe in their homes. Then there are other values that we don't agree on, and instead of accepting these value differences, we see others as "wrong." This creates an atmosphere in which we become more preoccupied with living with our "rightness" than having the space and grace for others whose values are different. That is a problem because whether we like the values of the woman sitting next to us, we share this planet and we need to be able to coexist. Enter *harmonious disagreement*.

Harmonious disagreement is a concept that comes from the experiences of Matteo Ricci, a sixteenth-century Jesuit priest and missionary to China. Imagine, if you will, a Catholic priest going to China to convert people to Christianity. Talk about an uphill battle. A country whose religious traditions included Indigenous folk religions, Confucianism, and Taoism, among others, now has a Catholic priest trying to convert people to follow a new, foreign religion. But Ricci and other Jesuits engaged in this endeavor, which is one of history's first recorded cross-cultural exchanges and the beginning of the dialogue between the East and the West.

Ricci didn't swoop in and start converting successfully; in fact, his efforts were largely unsuccessful. He faced many obstacles, including how he was perceived by others. There were language barriers, his foreign manner of dress, and his verbal and nonverbal comportment. Father Ricci was an alien to the Chinese citizens he met. What he had to do was to make friends with the scholars in his new country and attempt to create relationships in which there were stark value differences. So here's what he did: he engaged with his new acquaintances and friends on multiple subjects (like art, science, and philosophy), not just about spirituality and religion. He also adapted his practices to honor the culture in which he lived, such as changing the way he dressed to fit into his new country and remaining curious about his new home while also maintaining his values in a way that honored both. He conducted himself in alignment with his ethical beliefs, which transcended a particular doctrine, and was consistent in his treatment of others, no matter what values they held. There are lessons from Ricci's journey that are germane today and the basis for practicing harmonious disagreement.

The first lesson is that every individual is engaging in their evolution, and we must respect each other's journeys, even when they differ from our own. We can engage with each other in many ways, through a mutual enjoyment of talking, shared activities, and listening to each other's lived experiences. Even if we don't agree on everything, we can build and strengthen our relationships based on what we do have in common, so we have more solid ground when we talk about the things that we don't necessarily agree on. We can agree to disagree and still be respectful of each other. We can take responsibility for how our values may create impasses in our relationship and acknowledge that these impasses will cause some barriers in the relationship or put it at a standstill. Regardless of the impasse, we need to honor each other's perspective.

My favorite quote that illustrates the idea of harmonious disagreement comes from W. R. Purche, who said, "Everyone thinks they have the best dog. And none of them are wrong." This is a low-stakes example of how I will never be convinced that there is a pooch better than my Woodrow, and I know that other pet owners feel the same way about theirs. We can safely agree to disagree because their love of their pet doesn't threaten or take away from my love for mine. We can talk about our pets without the threat of a values war about who is the *best*. How might we use this example and bridge it out to other, more high-stakes values that we struggle to navigate in our social networks? Perhaps discourse about independence, freedom, work ethic, politics, or other topics that people value greatly? The sky is the limit.

ACCOUNTABILITY

One of the first ways we practice our values is to maintain our accountability to them in our social lives. This means taking responsibility for our actions and how they can impact our social connections, both IRL and in the virtual world. To a degree, accountability is the opposite of anonymity, because to be accountable and responsible, we must be known. Accountability in the virtual world is something that scholars have been wrestling with since its inception but without firm answers. This is because (in the United States) we are governed by the inherent right of free speech and freedom of expression, which can mean that I have a right to express myself even if it somehow hurts you or imposes on your feeling of safety or security. One example of the conflict between free speech and accountability comes from instances of hate speech and its impact on marginalized groups.

Here's a work-related example of my accountability in social settings. In this real-life example, I was called out by a colleague for something that I said about another colleague in our office. What I said wasn't appropriate or kind, and kindness is something that I value in my interactions. First off, I'm glad that I was called out about what I said, because I needed to be. Second, it's a great example of bystander intervention, where a third party intervenes on behalf of someone else who either isn't able or doesn't feel safe speaking up. In this instance, it was my job to take responsibility for what I said and to seek out the individual I offended in a private space to attempt to make amends and apologize.

Taking responsibility for your actions—no matter the modality—means that you have a clear understanding of your values, how you want to express those values, and the foresight to know that not everyone is going to share the same values as you. In my example, I was called out for violating my values, but there are some instances where I might be called out for violating a value that isn't as important to me. This is tricky, because when you find that you hold different values than others and your social network believes your values are too far from the commonly held social norms, they may try to correct you. Being sanctioned for expressing your values or your actions in the virtual world can be just as painful or embarrassing as it is in real life. Maybe even more so, because you're reading your scroll on your own, without anyone around for emotional support. If you're being sanctioned because your social network is trying to realign you with your values and you're acting outside of those values, this can be a good corrective interaction (like my real-life example). If your values don't align with your social group, this can cause conflict. Conflict isn't bad, but it's also an acknowledgment that we may differ on something important.

Another positive aspect of accountability is the unification of individuals under shared values that are prosocial, such as bystander intervention. Bystander intervention simply means that when you see something occurring, such as bullying, you call the bully out on their behavior as not appropriate or acceptable. A great example of this in social networks might be a group of women who mutually agree that gossip is not part of their culture; instead of tearing each other down, they speak positively about each other and with each other in virtual and real-life settings. If or when gossip occurs in this group, then members will call each other out and hold each other accountable for engaging in something that was identified as unacceptable.

The downside of accountability is that people can sometimes take it too far or attempt to overcorrect. Examples of this occur in popular culture when a celebrity posts an opinion that others don't agree with or like. Public shaming online is pervasive and the reason that so many virtual groups enforce community guidelines for their posts and comment sections. Shaming is the desire to humiliate an individual for what is perceived as their incorrect or bad behavior. It is an extreme version of sanction, designed to make someone feel "less than" and small. It can be very effective, and it can change how you feel about yourself. Continuous shaming is analogous to emotional abuse; think about that the next time you wade through gossip blogs or magazines. When I think about my interest in seeing which famous person is being torn down in the media, I must take responsibility and be accountable for the fact that I'm complicit in a machine designed to make someone else feel bad about themselves. It makes me feel ashamed of myself for being complicit in hurting someone else.

Further escalation of forced accountability is seen in the widely used practice of "cancel culture," which is the public boycotting or withdrawal of support for people, organizations, and so forth that are deemed unacceptable. The power here is in the group. Let's use an example those of us in midlife can remember from our early years. Remember the 1985 launch of New Coke? The mid-1980s was the height of the "cola wars," a cultural debate regarding whether Coke or Pepsi was the "best" soda. To distinguish itself, Coke developed a new product, colloquially called "New Coke." As I recall, New Coke was not well received, and it tasted terrible (early childhood memories being as reliable as they are). Consumers "canceled" New Coke: it remained unpurchased on store shelves, people didn't order it in restaurants, and consumers complained about it to the company. The power of cancel culture and the public is the reason we have Coca-Cola Classic today.

The middle school/"mean girls" example of canceling (which still happens today) occurs when a person is deemed "cool" and accepted, and then something happens, and they are suddenly "out." Cancel culture takes this a step further in that boycotting someone is akin to shunning and isolating them, which is emotionally abusive. Extreme behaviors in this case demonstrate a lack of compassion toward others and withholding forgiveness. Within our social connections, holding each other accountable can also mean narrowing our views about what is acceptable, to the point that many differences are excluded because they are deemed threatening. We see this when former family members are "canceled" through divorce. This exclusion can lead to increasing levels of division among people rather than unification, resulting in more polarization rather than meeting on common ground to explore what unites us.

ANONYMITY

Anonymity is the quality of being unknown and unrecognizable to others; this is a bit more challenging to pull off IRL. In the virtual world, anonymity occurs when we're able to use social platforms without using our legal names or identifiers to post to forums. Think Reddit. Anonymity in the virtual world is not assured in other social media platforms such as Instagram and Facebook, because users are required to use their legal names to sign up, authenticate through email, and so on. I think we all know this can be faked; ask a teenager. Engaging anonymously in the virtual world has been the subject of research for more than twenty years. In 2002, researchers were interested in how online communities could be anonymous while also holding individuals accountable to legal and moral standards that govern conduct

(Farkas et al., 2002). Fast forward to 2022, and researchers are still pondering these same questions but with more nuanced interpretations of what "anonymity" means. Scholars argue that anonymity is relative, given the relational nature of online communities and the complications associated therein with legal and ethical issues, technological advances, and social group affiliations, which can be inferred even when legal names are not (Eklund et al., 2022).

Moving around the virtual space anonymously to expand your social connections can be a liberating and fun way to learn about individuals, groups, and ideas that are different. You can wade into these new waters without leaving your comfort zone. Imagine something that you're curious about but aren't ready to say out loud to others; I guarantee there is a space for that somewhere in the virtual world. Much like accessibility enables us to make friends without navigating certain barriers, the relative anonymity of the virtual world allows us to satisfy our curiosity without great risk.

But there are downsides. Some folks enter unfamiliar spaces with an agenda that is more about judgment than curiosity. All of us are susceptible to this; my avatar on a social media platform or my anonymous handle on Reddit makes me faceless, or less human. The same can be said for others who are engaged in virtual space. Engaging in cruelty and other hurtful behaviors becomes easier when we are disembodied and don't view each other as "real." In real-life interactions with people, we can see their facial and bodily reactions to the things that we say and do; those "nonverbals" provide the clues we need to know when we've hurt them. Reading nonverbals and experiencing the reactions to the things we say is also part of limbic resonance and allows us to experience empathy for others. This is lessened or nonexistent when we're online and can't anticipate or see another person's response.

Another downside is deindividuation, which can happen when we associate with online groups. Deindividuation is the process by which individuals lose their sense of individual identity and digress into antisocial behavior or submit to group mentality, sometimes referred to as "mob mentality." Being part of a group can be a good thing, but it depends on the group. Pretend that you want to join a virtual group of strong, independent midlife women. Now let's pretend that as you get more engaged online, you begin to see messages within the group that being a strong, independent midlife woman means that you see asking for help from others (especially men) as a weakness. Other women post examples of how their friends or partners offer support, and the online group turns negative: "This isn't being a strong, independent midlife woman!" You read these messages and eventually start to buy into this mentality in a way that you hadn't before; you believe in getting support, but maybe if these other women you admire are saying this is the way to be strong, then you'd better hop on the bus.

This may seem like a silly example, but it illustrates how you can get sucked into thinking like a group rather than living by your own beliefs and values. It also explains how people in groups can become bolder and more aggressive; the cover of the group gives them the anonymity to say and do things they normally wouldn't do. This can happen IRL or online, but with the expansion of online groups, it is easier to be anonymous in these forums. We see more serious and extreme affiliation in online hate groups, which propagate the notion that certain people are "bad" or "dangerous." The organizational power that groups can marshal is very similar to the daily "two-minute hate" described in George Orwell's *1984*, in which citizens unite daily to shout and express anger toward the government's endorsed enemy. Within the group, citizens share emotions and vent frustration toward a mutual enemy, but very few stop to question why they are expressing hate or if it is necessarily healthy or good. This can become a danger of group membership if we don't engage in self-reflection.

ACCESSIBILITY

The final *A* is the most familiar to us: the overall accessibility of our social networks to us through the physical technology that we have that helps us to connect. We can access our social networks through our computers, phones, smartwatches, and other devices, which are typically within easy reach. Getting into contact with our social networks IRL is more challenging without using technology; seeing all our IRL people frequently isn't something many of us can do. Not only does technology and the virtual world make it easy for us to get connected, but it can also help make communication far more transactional than ever before. A great example comes from my older sister who wanted a recipe from a friend. She commented that she needed a measurement for something that she was making and decided to text her friend because, "It's so much easier, I don't have to get into a conversation, I can just get what I need and get on with my day." I don't disagree that it is a huge benefit, but at the same time, isn't it interesting that our lives may feel so busy or our schedules so tight that we don't have the space for a three-minute conversation while obtaining flour measurements for a friend's cake recipe?

Much like the example of my sister's transactional use of texting, easy access to our social networks makes it possible for us to stay up to date with people who are far away. We can access their lives through social media, use real-time video chats to stay connected, and share texts and memes at our leisure. It's also way cheaper than it used to be. When I was a kid, I remember my mom making long-distance phone calls to her twin sister on the other side of the country almost every day. I remember my father and mother's conversations about the cost of long-distance phone calls and trying to get the best deals from carriers (wow—that's a blast from the past). Now we can call and connect at a flat rate, which also includes high-speed internet access and unlimited connection. Cost no longer limits us to communicating only for special occasions (like calling long-distance or to foreign countries was in the old days), but at the same time, do we take advantage of these cost-effective ways to connect? Or are we like my sister, just trying to get the information that we need amid the pressure of our daily lives?

Another huge benefit of accessibility is that it can put people in touch with each other, especially those with special interests or in unique circumstances. For individuals who struggle with high levels of social anxiety, online communities can provide a way to connect that feels safer. For individuals in rural areas who may be isolated due to physical location or interest, online communities offer an opportunity to feel less alone and to help overcome the barrier of transportation and time to go to a larger town. Online also can be a way to connect when your life circumstances have changed and limit your ability to get out. I think about when I was helping to care for my father at the end of his life. My only connection with my social supports was through virtual forums, and I am grateful that I had them! Another example comes from a midlife woman who was struggling to connect while navigating severe and persistent mental health issues and co-occurring health issues. Her ability to find an online community, build a support network, and provide support to her fellow group members was invaluable in her journey of self-acceptance and social connectedness. Without these avenues to access people with relative ease, our lives likely would have been much smaller.

The downside of this accessibility to our networks can include the ubiquity of the technology and our availability if we choose to engage. Most ladies I know always have their phones in hand and feel as if they're missing an appendage if they don't have it with them. Unless we create and maintain clear boundaries around our access to our social networks, we can get sucked into being connected almost 24/7, without an opportunity for breaks. And this can happen without us being cognizant of it.

We get a chemical payout from checking our phones, basically a dopamine hit in our brains, a reward that is like the experience we have after exercising, sex, eating food, or having a positive social interaction. While we are seeking the dopamine hit of connection, we're being rewarded for checking our tech; this positive reward leads us to repeatedly check our phones. But our brain is smart. It knows that while it is getting the chemical release, it isn't receiving the deeper connection that engaging with others IRL (limbic resonance) can give. Unfortunately, social media and cell phones were designed to exploit our natural dopamine reward centers, and this savvy use of our animalistic nature can have the negative impact of making us crave the very thing that makes us feel less connected (Haynes & Clements, 2018).

Chemical payoff is one of the reasons that individuals can lack boundaries around their technology. What constitutes healthy boundaries for one person can be very different than what it means for others; boundaries exist on a continuum. As midlife women, we may find that our attention is diverted in several different ways: children, partners, work, aging parents, social networks, and so on. For example, letting your friends know that you need to keep your technology readily accessible when your kids go out for the night to ensure that they can get in touch with you if needed is a healthy boundary. However, if you're out with friends and tell them that you want to be fully present but you spend half the evening checking your phone messages and work emails when it isn't necessary, it likely will be perceived as disrespectful. Your boundaries are only as good as (1) you're able to communicate about them and (2) you're able to maintain them. In the first example, your friends have context and understand your boundaries and will respect them; in the second, you said one thing, but your behaviors are the opposite, and your friends' perception of how you value your relationship likely will change.

Sometimes our lack of boundaries comes from one of the most insidious ways that technology and accessibility capture the interest of our dopamine receptors: *the notification*. Notifications can be so handy in alerting us to new messages or calls that are waiting for our response. Not only is it a reward, but it also can create a sense of obligation to be readily available, to respond quickly, to be involved and on top of things. I think that the combination of dopamine rewards, internalized pressure to be available, people-pleasing, and constant pinging from notifications can sometimes drive our fear of missing out (FOMO).

The final downside that I discuss here is the haunting nature of information that lives in the virtual world that will never go away; it will always be accessible. This can happen without our consent (posts that are created about us that we have no control over) and with our consent (the post that seemed like a good idea at the time, but in a different light does not reflect well on us). By the time we reach our middle years, that could be a great deal of information about us that is out in the world and that may not be reflective of the people we are today. The choices I made as a younger woman are not the choices I would make today; I cringe thinking about the existence of an online scrapbook of those decisions for my future employers, social acquaintances, and frenemies to Google and find. The lesson here is to enjoy the accessibility of your social networks and to consider what and how you share, because it will impact you today and tomorrow.

FINDING BALANCE IN OUR SOCIAL LIVES

The question that continues to circle my mind in all this information is how do we find the right balance for ourselves? Having and maintaining your social circle is an important part of your overall well-being, and there are many factors to consider. When our values conflict with people in our social circles, we may want to consider how the tenets of harmonious disagreement can help us to accept what we cannot change about others and encourage us to remain civil with each other. Maintaining our accountability to ourselves in our relationships with others is ultimately our job, but if we have friends who call us out when we behave poorly, we can evaluate our actions and correct them when needed. When we navigate our virtual social worlds and real-life social connections, we may oscillate between being anonymous and being known—do we act the same way in each place? The answer we give to that question may be revealing. Last, how much access to our social connections is enough? Each of us experiences our need for social connection on a continuum, and the bandwidth we have can change over time. Factors to consider when accessing and assessing your social health can include the balance between real-life and virtual connection, your accessibility to your social circle, and reconciling your need for being known and/or privacy with how you engage with your social networks. The reflection questions below can help you consider your social health and engagement, allowing you to evaluate where you are now and if it meets where you want to be.

REFLECTION QUESTIONS

- What are your values for social interactions—whether online or face-to-face?
- How do you feel after face-to-face interactions versus social media interactions? What is satisfying or unsatisfying about those interactions?
- Are there ways you get your social needs met online in ways that you can't in your current real-life community?
- Are there communities you want to explore online that you might not want or be able to in face-to-face communities?

- What rules do you have for yourself in your online interactions that keep you functioning within your values in the same way you do with real-life interactions?
- What boundaries do you have for your social interactions (real life or online)?
- What boundaries do you want to have?
- How do you maintain accountability for these boundaries (e.g., an accountability partner, using notifications, app limits for screen-time, downtime)?

CHAPTER EIGHT

VOCATION

Sitting with a professional colleague at a conference, we talked about our careers. Each of us had been in our respective fields for around fifteen to twenty years at this point, and we were questioning if the motives that had brought us to the field were the same ones that were keeping us here. She remarked that her mom had posted a meme on her Facebook page about her career: "If the ladder is not leaning against the right wall, every step we take just gets us to the wrong place faster." But how can we tell the difference between a rough patch and the wrong wall?

This conversation happened at an interesting time in my career. I am the queen of working multiple jobs simultaneously; even today people ask me, "How many jobs do you have now?" It used to be a funny joke, but now I think of it as a sad reflection about how I've bought into "busyness" culture and function out of fear that if I don't make myself irreplaceable, I'll be replaced. This fear came to life while conversing with a former provost at my institution, when it came up that I was completely replaceable. I was shocked and hurt. I had spent a great deal of time working very hard in two different offices on my campus for them to be successful, to the point of imbalance in my personal life. Rather than being given words of praise or affirmation, I was being told that, to my hearing, it didn't matter what I did, because they could find someone else to do the same thing—that was how the world worked. As I reflect, I wonder if this individual believed that he was offering me some kind of sage life lesson that would help me be successful or better balanced or if he was simply being callous. Regardless of his intent, the encounter left its mark.

I still work at the same university, but my work duties have changed. I hold a position with more focused responsibilities than I had in the past, and I'm fortunate that I have the autonomy to make decisions about the work that I do (within reason). Working on this book is an example of my autonomy; I've made it part of what I do so that I can find fulfillment in my work; some of my other roles lacked the same level of satisfaction. Thinking back on these conversations with peers and administrators, the intervening years prompted me to wonder if my job was the place where I was going to find fulfillment. And if it wasn't, did I need to stop exhausting myself to find fulfillment where I wasn't going to receive it? I also had to look more broadly at the vocation I chose to determine if it was still my calling or if I needed to be brave and find a new "wall."

That's what we discuss in this chapter: what vocation is, how we may experience exhaustion or burnout from our job, and how to reconceptualize the place that work and career have in our lives. Keep in mind that your *vocation* (what you do with your life that makes you feel fulfilled and whole, your life's purpose) isn't necessarily your *job* (the activity that earns you money).

VOCATION IS WHAT YOU DO

Vocation has several definitions, but the one that I use to guide this chapter is "a person's employment or main occupation, especially regarded as particularly worthy and requiring great dedication" (Merriam-Webster.com). What is particularly important about this definition is the distinction between "employment" and "occupation." Employment (job) is often thought of as what we do for our job and to get the money that we need to live our lives. Occupation, on the other hand, can be considered a way of spending time. You may or may not make money from the activities that occupy you, but they can be intrinsically rewarding and satisfying. Internal satisfaction from certain occupations can make them important to you regardless of the external rewards that you may receive from them. As children and young adults, we're encouraged to "do what you love and you'll never work a day in your life." However, it doesn't always happen that way. When there is misalignment between what we love and what pays the bills, it can be hard to stay motivated. Another scenario involves falling out of love with what we chose to do in our earlier lives and wondering what our next steps are. This a common issue of many midlife women with whom I work, and it has caused them to reevaluate their careers and vocations.

When my book coach read this chapter, she noted, "In midlife, we often get tired and want to stab our own eyeballs out; work gets stale." Upon reflection, the comment seems both accurate and dramatic. I don't know that I've been in a place of wanting to stab my eyeballs out, but I can relate to the frustration of feeling as though my daily work is no longer novel, interesting, impactful, or challenging. Yes, unique scenarios arise that provide me an opportunity to think in a new way, but once you've figured out how to do your job well over time, those scenarios feel few and far between. One insight that I've recognized recently is that keeping my work life interesting is up to me, which can be challenging depending on how much autonomy I have in my work. I bet the same is true for you.

Some ladies who read this chapter love what they do. To you, I say: I envy you. You have found happiness in marrying your employment and occupation in a way that still fulfills you. Many of us strive for that level of contentment: we want to be you when we grow up. Along the spectrum of vocational satisfaction, some put work on autopilot, doing what needs to be done and leaving work at work. The women in these careers know that their work provides a level of satisfaction, and although it may not be completely fulfilling, they are content with their jobs and keep doing what they are doing with less frustration or restlessness than others may feel.

I confess that I also envy these women. I have tried to improve my ability to compartmentalize my work and to remain satisfied with work that is stable, but the striving part of me fights against this contentment. And then there are those who experience a sense of restlessness with their work, which prevents them from feeling satisfied. The origins of these feelings can arise from a lack of mental stimulation, a toxic work culture, or stress due being overburdened at work and beyond, being underpaid and underrecognized, experiencing burnout, or no longer being suited to what we once did (i.e., falling out of love) and casting about to find what will make us feel more fulfilled.

Here's the thing about our vocation: it's how we contribute to the world in our unique way. The hope is that, although we are replaceable, what we want and need is to be able to engage in work that gives us meaning and a sense of purpose. In existential terms, "a vocation means nothing but such a direction of life activities as renders them perceptibly significant to a person, because of the consequences they accomplish, and also useful to his associates" (Dewey, 1916, as cited in Higgins, 2005). As Dewey states, we need to feel that what we do is significant, and it's a nice bonus if what we do is helpful to others. This motivates many of the women with whom I work: that what they do matters and that the purpose, value, and impact extend beyond themselves. In addition to the existential value of work, research also shows that women who work in midlife enjoy better health later in life, not only because of the benefits derived from income, but also the inherent meaning and social connections that a workplace can provide (Caputo, Pavalko, & Hardy, 2020).

Thinking along these lines, we explore your overall vocational satisfaction and how burnout may play into how you experience your work life in this chapter. We also explore tools that can help you to put your job in its "place" in your life, despite a culture that tells us that what we do is one of our most important characteristics. Finally, we discuss finding fulfillment while balancing the need to pay the bills and how these tasks can align in a way that can help us to experience greater vocational satisfaction. First, let's see what percentage of your focus work takes in your overall life.

WORK-LIFE BALANCE PIE CHART EXERCISE

One of my favorite exercises to use when women are trying to determine how much focus their vocation receives is to have them complete a pie chart. With this exercise, you divide a typical circle in terms of how much time and energy certain parts of your life receive. This activity is a departure from previous chapter exercises, but the amount of time we put into certain endeavors reflects the value that we place on them. With this idea in mind, we look at our values in a slightly different way here.

The example shown in figure 8.1 was completed by my friend Simpa as part of an interview for this chapter. Much like Simpa, you may ask, what goes on the pie chart? You should include whatever is important to you and that you spend time and energy doing. Through our chat, she determined that the main foci in her life are work (note that for Simpa "work" and "vocation" are the same; this is not true for everyone), hobbies, personal growth, caring for the family pets, and helping to care for her parents. You can see her pie chart in figure 8.1.

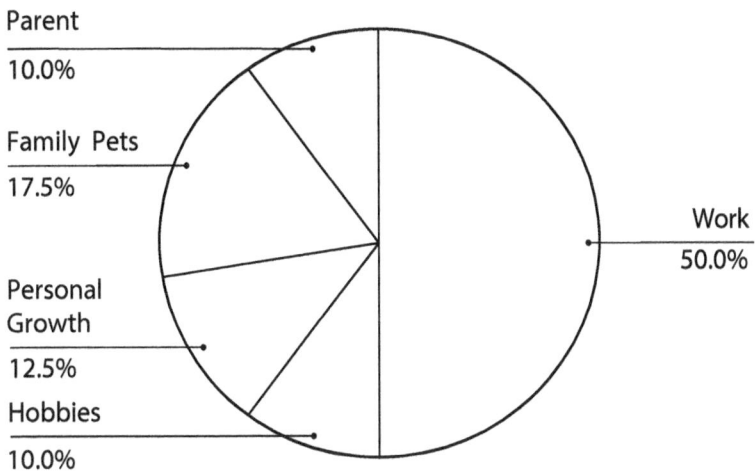

Figure 8.1. Simpa's Work-Life Balance Pie Chart

Now it's your turn. Using figure 8.2, create a breakdown of how much time your work and vocation receive compared to the rest of your life and obligations. I recommend using a pencil in case you need to make changes as you read through the chapter. Remember that, unlike Simpa's example, your work and your vocation may not be the same thing.

As you read this chapter, think about how your pie chart represents the balance of your vocational and work life with the rest of your life. We're going to tackle challenging issues, like burnout and keeping your vocational/work life as a part of your life rather than your whole life. You may find that you need to adjust your percentages as you read through some of the indicators that I discuss, and that's fine. This is a snapshot of how you believe your work is impacting you right now.

Figure 8.2. Your Work-Life Balance Pie Chart

BURNOUT

About five years ago I took a burnout inventory to gauge if I was experiencing this issue at work. I thought I was because I had some classic symptoms: I was exhausted, I engaged in a lot of cynical humor and sarcasm, and I didn't think that the work that I was doing mattered. At that time in my career, it felt like high tide: the waves were cresting, and they just kept coming, with no relief in sight. According to the assessment, the factor that categorized me as experiencing "work distress" rather than burnout was my resilience, because I also experienced a high level of satisfaction from my work, despite feeling as though I was moving a beach one grain of sand at a time. I felt very invalidated by that result; it left me questioning how much worse I had to feel before I met the criteria for burnout (at least for this assessment).

The World Health Organization (WHO) defines burnout as "a syndrome conceptualized as resulting from chronic workplace stress that has not been successfully managed" (WHO, 2019). Not only did the

WHO define it, but it also created a code for it in the International Classifications of Disease (ICD) catalog as an occupational phenomenon (not a medical condition). The definition raised some questions for me. Who is supposed to be successfully managing this chronic stress? Is this only my job? Is it my employer's job? Are we in this together? In the United States, we value rugged individualism and independence; however, burnout speaks to a systemic issue that pervades organizations and impacts the people in them. To me, it feels as though burnout is a systemic issue that we must each individually solve on our own, often with less than satisfactory results.

Why Are We Experiencing Burnout?

During our midlife years, we play a very important role in the dynamics of our organizations. Typically, we have more institutional knowledge or maturity (or both) than our younger coworkers and are highly engaged in our careers when compared to our older coworkers (Infurna, Gerstorf, & Lachman, 2020). Midlife workers tend to play a role in both nurturing their coworkers and creating a bridge between younger and older generations, similar to the role that we play in our private lives. For those of us who are experiencing our midlife years at this point in history, we are also part of a society in which fewer children are being born and our aging population is increasing, which makes those in midlife an important resource to current society (Infurna et al., 2023). The phenomenon of being in the middle—also known as the sandwich generation—puts a great deal of pressure on Gen X and millennials to support those who belong to older and younger generational cohorts.

For these reasons and others, many women whom I counsel experience work burnout in their midlife years. Studies show that variables that can contribute to burnout include work environments that are highly demanding and that offer low levels of social support and control (Soares, Grossi, & Sundin, 2007). Coupling high-demand jobs with other issues, such as outside caregiving responsibilities and/or chronic health concerns, it is reasonable that women experience burnout due to increasing demands and not enough social support to manage them. These demands and the resulting symptoms of burnout may be why we see a gender gap in the number of sick days that women take compared to their male counterparts (Østby, Mykletun, & Nilsen, 2018).

   I don't know about you, but it seems as if every year I'm being asked to do even more at work than the previous year with either the same resources or shrinking ones. As we experienced after the pandemic, rising prices and inflation impact the cost of everything, making it more challenging for businesses to operate and for us to operate our lives with the same resources. The mental gymnastics of managing an increased workload on a shoestring while simultaneously managing life with fewer resources is hard. Another circumstance that leads to burnout is the feeling that we lack time; because of additional tasks at work, we can sometimes feel as though we don't have time to complete the things that we need to. Sometimes these tasks are assigned by our superiors and sometimes they are situations that we create for ourselves. For example, while researching this book at my academic office, I didn't close my door, and even though coworkers and students could see that my desk was covered with articles, they stopped by to ask questions or catch up as they walked down the hall. Don't get me wrong: the relationships I have with my students and coworkers are one of the best parts of my job. My later frustration about not getting my research done in the time allotted was the direct result of my lack of boundaries: I hadn't created the boundary of closing the door so that I could work undisturbed. Things that we can't control (our bosses' demands) and things we choose not to control (closing the door to ensure quiet for the task at hand) both contribute to burnout. As I thought about the reasons that midlife women experience burnout, I came up with a short list of the main reasons that I've seen in my practice, which include:

- *Emotional labor.* As discussed, midlife workers tend to be invaluable resources in their organizations. Women often are asked to engage in more emotional labor (to nurture coworkers) than their male counterparts. The problem with providing emotional labor in the workplace is that it often translates into "nonpromotable work," meaning these tasks aren't going to help you move forward in your career and often can detract from work you could be doing to move forward in your career. Ultimately, such work may benefit the organization, but unless your organization sees this work as important and a reason to move you forward in the company, it will not help you achieve your personal career goals.

- *Work-life balance.* Many women I speak with have a hard time turning work off during their downtime. This may be due to internalized pressure, messages from their organization to meet work needs at all times, and/or a culture that prizes busyness. No matter the reason, not having clear boundaries between work and the rest of your life can mean that you never have the opportunity to turn off your work brain. This lack of rest can lead to fatigue and burnout.
- *High demands in the workplace.* With constant demands on our time, tight deadlines for projects, multiple simultaneous projects (which scatters our focus), and/or large workloads with limited resources or support, we are primed to become overwhelmed.
- *Limited career advancement opportunities/underrepresentation in leadership roles.* Although we have made great strides as working women, the reality is that there is still a great deal of disparity between men's and women's opportunities in the workplace. Being overlooked for additional training and promotions, unequal pay, and not seeing other women in leadership roles or a clear path to growing into leadership roles can cause disillusionment and resentment at work.
- *Lack of support in the work environment.* This can range from feeling unsupported at work, not having mentors to help answer questions, to experiencing discrimination and sexism. Any of these issues can make going to work hard. Add to this a range of issues, which can include ongoing microaggressions to overt discrimination. These aggressions can create a toxic environment that is poisonous to the soul.
- *Double-shift syndrome.* Many women are still responsible for the bulk of caregiving and household chores after their full-time job ends for the day. A never-ending cycle of job/caregiving/chores, day in and day out, is a recipe for exhaustion.

Responses to Burnout

Although this doesn't list every reason that a midlife woman may experience burnout, it's a good representation of some of the common concerns that may resonate with you. When we experience work fatigue and burnout, we may attempt to "push through." Sometimes we push until we realize that we can't push any longer, and our minds and bodies give valuable clues that it's time to stop pushing and pay attention to ourselves. Embodied experiences of burnout can be chronic illness, fatigue, looping negative thoughts, lowered self-esteem and self-concept, feeling like a failure in one or multiple areas of your life, withdrawal from activities you love, depression, and anxiety.

"Quiet quitting" is a phenomenon that gained attention around 2022, when pandemic employees did the required minimum at work while silently looking for other employment (Hare, 2022). We all have had times when we needed to do the minimum at work because of life obligations, but this went deeper. It was a chronic level of disengagement at work. I see this on two sides (and I'm sure there are more). As a supervisor, I know that quiet quitting can bring down the whole team because coworkers ultimately fill the gap created by the person doing the minimum. As a person who has had spaces in my life where I did the minimum at work, it was what I needed to do to pay my bills and keep my head above water while going through a bad time.

Quiet quitting doesn't happen in a vacuum, and it often coincides with other negative work behaviors that worsen feelings of burnout. These can include over-engaging in negative conversations and gossip at work (raises hand guiltily), overworking to get ahead (there will always be more work; it is a never-ending well), projecting negative thoughts and intentions onto others (typically those in power), and blaming others for your experience of burnout. It also includes looking at your job with a negativity bias, losing sight of the positive aspects that exist within your work. Don't get me wrong: if you're in a toxic work environment, I am not asking you to engage in toxic positivity (i.e., pretending that everything is fine and ignoring the real problems that exist in your workplace). However, if you only actively pay attention to the negative aspects of your work, you may be missing on the good and positive ones.

When mired in burnout, we likely experience lowered levels of self-worth. This lowered sense of worth can leave us doubting ourselves, our purpose, and our vocational choices. What if we view our lowered sense of self-worth as an opportunity to take a step back and see what impact our vocation has on our overall lives? This is a powerful move away from thinking that lowered self-worth indicates that we are somehow burnt out because we are failing. I say this because what I hear from women suffering burnout is that they feel as if they are not doing enough or have failed when often the opposite is true. These women are doing too much; the "failure" (if it can be called that) is that their work and vocational lives have encroached too far into the rest of their lives.

Many women expect that their vocation is tied to their purpose, which contributes to feelings of self-worth. Sometimes our workplace isn't where we're going to find this sense of purpose. Remember that our purpose or vocation is a higher calling that matters to us and may not be found within our work lives. When we are overwhelmed with factors that can increase our susceptibility to burnout, we can lose sight of why we do what we do. To maintain our affinity for our vocation and purpose, I think it can be helpful to think about how we can put our vocation in its place, decentering it from one of our main foci to one of the things that we do in our lives. (*She says as she continues to struggle to do this very thing every day.*)

Let's try this together.

PUTTING OUR VOCATION IN ITS PLACE

While rethinking my relationship to my work, I came up with this question that helped catalyze how I think about my career: *if I am replaceable in my job, how can I replace my job as the main focal point of my vocational life?* Yes, our work is important, but engaging in work that feels less satisfying or unfulfilling means that we need to take a step back and reframe how we think about our vocational journey. This forced me to revisit a question I posed earlier in the chapter: *whose job is it to help me prevent burnout and remain satisfied with my vocation?* It's mine because no one else cares about this issue as much as I do.

Around this time, I had a conversation with a colleague and friend who has worked as an administrative supervisor at a mental health facility for many years. She was experiencing burnout and decided to do something amazing: she asked for a sabbatical. Because she had longevity at her work and social capital with her executive leadership, she was able to take several months off to refresh and rethink her career. Though this is not an opportunity available to all of us, I think we can all benefit from her insights. She shared with me that one of the best things that she did was to rethink how she was designing her overall life and her work life.

Many of her insights were inspired by reading *Designing Your Work Life* (Burnett & Evans, 2021), a book that I highly recommend reading in its entirety. The authors are designers by trade, and many of the ways that they work through problems and find solutions are how counselors are taught to help clients. They utilize a tool that therapists also use often: reframes. A reframe is a way of looking at a problem differently than you have already approached it; it means taking a step back to consider other viewpoints. An example of a problem might be, "I have too much to do and will never get everything done." Reframing the problem might be, "How can I create a hierarchy of my most important work tasks and use a priority list to manage my time?"

Reframing requires flexibility in the ways that we think about problems, which can feel challenging because we may feel stuck. However, stepping outside of our tightly held assumptions about our jobs and seeing how they may be holding us hostage is a useful exercise. I have found that the assumptions that I hold about my work are only held by me and no one else. I think it's a powerful insight that I am often the person who is putting restrictions on me in my work life. For example, when I was trying to be more flexible in evaluating the value of my vocation and work, I started to ask myself the question, *"How can I make my job work for me?"* This was an interesting way for me to think about my work: That it and I are in a reciprocal relationship. Not that I worked for my job, but it also needed to work for me. Reframing my relationship with my work has helped me to consider ways that I wasn't making my job work for me and ways that it could.

While I was becoming more flexible in my thinking, another nugget that helped me was Burnett and Evans's (2021) ideas regarding metrics that can be used to measure success. They discuss ways that they have found that can help individuals measure their success and can allow for some balance in how they approach their work life. The three main measures they propose are money, impact, and expression. Money is exactly what sounds like: the amount of money you make in your job and how important money is to you at a given point in your life. Impact is how your work creates a difference or change in the world. Again, this is a place to be flexible in your thinking, because all work has the potential to be impactful. For example, if you're a real estate agent, your impact is helping people find a new home or business location, which is very important. Expression is how your work or occupation allows you to be creative and what you bring to the world that is unique to you. I believe that some think that creativity is limited to those who are in the arts, but I have seen creative thinking and solutions in a variety of careers and job settings.

What I like about these metrics and the way that the authors present them is that you can adapt each of them to your life in a way that makes sense for you. If you have a family and a lot of bills that need to be paid, then money may be your highest metric of success. However, it isn't the only metric. You can also look at how your occupation contributes to your impact and expression. For example, an individual who is a financial planner may make a good deal of money (highest priority metric), and she knows that by helping others plan for their retirement, she is making a huge impact on individuals around her now and in the future (second-highest-priority metric). Although the expression metric isn't her highest priority, she takes pride in understanding different investment portfolios and putting together strategies that meet the needs of the individuals she works with. She uses her knowledge, skills, and judgment to create a plan of action that is unique to her experience.

You'll notice that I've used the impact metric throughout this chapter. I've done so because most of the women with whom I work believe that impact is one of the highest values that their vocation holds for them. However, these metrics for success may not be the ones that you hold for yourself. Consider substituting your values for your work/vocational life for the metrics discussed in this section. How do you embody these values in your vocational life?

How Will This Help You Put Your Job in Its Place?

True confession: so far, this has been the hardest chapter of this book to write. Why? Because this is the area of my life that I go to therapy for. My equilibrium between work and the rest of my life is not always appropriately balanced. It wasn't always this way; my ability to balance work and life changed when I started my doctoral program. I was living in a new city, without friends or family around, and my focus was being successful in this big, important degree program. Here's the thing about people in higher education: for the most part, they like to get A's. Except, at some point, there are no more grades to earn, but people still strive for invisible grades or benchmarks. Higher education isn't any different from other career paths in that there are specific things that you must do to maintain your job and get promoted. The difference is that a confluence of smart people are actively pursuing being "the best" well past the point where making metaphorical A's should be the metric for success.

Possibly I am projecting onto my peers; however, my observations suggest I am not far from the truth. How can my struggle help you? In the last few years, I have tried hard to get an A in "putting my job in its place"; I have tried many things that I share with you here in the hopes that some of these can work for you. Also, I have failed, a lot, in putting my work in its place, hence the therapy. I say this to you to normalize that it's okay if your work overtakes your life sometimes too. Tomorrow is a new day for us all to restart and create better boundaries around our work lives. Let's get started with some of the ways that you can work to keep your job in its place as part of your life, not the focus of your life.

- *Set boundaries.* What are the hard lines around your work that you don't cross? What are the more permeable boundaries that you've let slide that you need to strengthen? A few years ago, on a vacation, my partner asked that I turn off the work email app on my phone. It was a game changer—no more insistent dinging on my phone after hours or on vacation. This is a boundary I've maintained for years that has helped me control my "Pavlov's dog" response to emails. What boundaries do you need to enforce?
- *Practice time management.* First, let me say that it isn't a time management issue if you have too much to do at work and not enough

time to do it. That is an unrealistic expectation issue that we talk about in a few bullets. However, managing your work time when you have the autonomy to do so is important. There are times in my days/weeks that don't belong to me (mandatory meetings) and others that do. How I plan the time that I do control is important. For example, I set a timer on my phone and answer emails during a forty-five-minute block in the morning. This way, I've triaged communication, responded in a timely manner to most folks, and addressed one of my primary work responsibilities during a time and space that works for me. The email flow doesn't stop, but practicing this time management skill changes my response to the flow.

- *Say no.* The work FOMO is real, but you don't have to buy in. As women, I think we're conditioned to say yes because (1) it's nice, (2) it's expected, (3) we're not always taught to discern which tasks are beneficial to us versus beneficial to our organizations and that are not going to help us in the long run. The best advice I've ever gotten about saying yes or no to anything: ask for at least twenty-four hours to consider your answer, determine how this task benefits your career in a meaningful way, and determine what work task you will let go in order to take on the new task. When you practice these skills in a meaningful way, it's a game changer.
- *Communicate with your employer.* Ugh, why is this so uncomfortable? However, communicating what you need to your employer is (hopefully) a way for you to manage both your and their expectations for how you manage your work life. Being clear about your boundaries in an overt way (i.e., communicating them) versus a covert way (i.e., not being explicit about your boundaries; leaving people to guess) is one of the better ways to set expectations for what you can and will do in your work life. For example, this is one of the places where you can communicate unrealistic work expectations. (Let me also say that in my experience this can be an ongoing process if your higher-ups are less responsive to helping.) One of the best resources I have found lately for communicating work boundaries comes from Melissa Urban's *The Book of Boundaries* (New York: Dial Press). She gives great, easy-to-follow

examples of dialogue you can use in work settings. I've used it and have recommended it to friends and clients.
- *Manage your work/collegial relationships.* In the last chapter, I gave an example of a social relationship at work that was rocky and around which I needed to create some boundaries. Your work/collegial relationships will run the spectrum, from folks you really like who may be close friends to those you interact with simply as a point of doing business. Part of keeping your work in its place is knowing the limits of these relationships and how carrying these relationships into your private life may impact how you disconnect from work (if that is your goal).
- *Unplug regularly.* News that's not news: your brain gets tired and needs to rest. Unplugging from your work life allows you to recharge, refresh, and gives your brain time to process problems and challenges (often unbeknownst to you, but that's a bit of brain magic). Unplugging from work can mean turning off email notifications, taking time away (vacation time, a mental health day, whatever), and being present in your off time to do what you need to recharge (hanging with friends and family, trying a new recipe, skydiving). But planning to do it regularly is important. For example, you could create a plan to take one mental health day every two months. You may find that it helps you to recharge, rest, and manage your work life differently.

Building boundaries around our work to keep it in its place can take a lot of time, energy, trial, and error. What works today may not work next week, and so much of it is dependent upon whom you're working with. In an ideal world, you are in a work and vocational environment that gives you the autonomy and flexibility to build the life that you want, but that is not the case for many. For this reason, I recommend starting small with one step. For me, it began with turning off the email app on my phone; for you, it may be something different. The question is, what is the most important place for you to begin so that you can feel some success in decentering your vocational life as a focus? The next section briefly discusses and normalizes feelings of wanting to walk away and quit your job.

USING THE ESCAPE HATCH: WE'VE ALL FANTASIZED ABOUT IT

Our vocation and work are important, whether they are the same or two different things for you; we know that our vocation is a way that we create meaning and purpose in our lives, working in midlife can aid us in aging well, can give us stability in terms of money and benefits, and is one of the identities that we carry. But sometimes work doesn't feel like it's going to work anymore.

This section is not a call to "quiet quit" or to participate in the second coming of the Great Resignation; rather, it is to normalize that we have all *wanted* to quit (Gittleman, 2022). Some of us have had the opportunity to do so, either by necessity or opportunity. When it is necessary, it may be due to health or mental health reasons, and you simply cannot continue to work in the same place or in the same capacity as you have previously. The other side of the coin can be that you have an opportunity to leave a vocation or job by your own choice to pursue a new job opening or a completely different career path. This is an exciting opportunity that also can be exhilarating and scary at the same time. Here's the thing about fantasy: you control the narrative without the consequences of real-life implications. This is an important distinction when you imagine leaving your work versus when you actually leave and must manage the consequences (positive and negative) of doing so.

In my interview with Simpa, she shared a story about a particularly hard time at her work. There was an organizational change, and her new supervisor was a micromanager. She was, for a time, the focus of this manager's ire, and it seemed as though she couldn't do anything right. This loss of autonomy and feeling as though she was mistrusted by her direct superior caused her a great deal of distress. Although Simpa didn't necessarily have to work past her typical hours, the emotional turmoil bled into her time with her family, her weekends, and invaded her thoughts when she wanted to focus on other things.

She laughed as she shared the story about how she had called her financial planner to find out what would happen if she cashed out her retirement savings and just quit. The penalties were prohibitive, and the reality was that she was not going to do it, but as she said, "I just needed to ask the question to explore my options. Sometimes when it's bad, I need to know that I have choices." Simpa's story is like many of ours: she manages her work life and does her best, but the reality is that there are times when work conditions aren't ideal. And just like most of us, she needs her job to earn money. Returning to the metrics proposed by Burnett and Evans, Simpa identified that money was the main reason that she maintained her job. Although she enjoys the impact she has at her company and she finds ways to express herself outside of her job, she knows that as a woman in the world, she needs her job so that she can live and thrive. In her search for other work, she hasn't found another job that satisfies her needs nor is the work landscape currently favorable to her skill set and work environment preferences. In other words, for now, she feels stuck. For Simpa, using boundaries to keep her work in its place in her life is imperative to maintaining her level of satisfaction with her overall life and vocation.

Another individual I worked with, Cass, had to leave her vocation out of necessity due to physical and mental health problems. Cass had to take a step back from the world of work to continue to survive. Due to illness, managing her symptoms became a full-time job, which didn't allow her the time or energy to engage in her vocation in the same way that she once did. This was not an escape, but rather felt like the betrayal of her body, one that took her a long time to come to terms with. For Cass, this also meant that vocation wasn't something she could put her full energy into nor was it something that she could depend on for income. In Cass's case, she ended up in a long battle to win disability benefits. What she found at that time was that she still needed to engage in what she felt was her vocation but in a different way. For Cass, teaching was how she found meaning. She continued expanding her knowledge of what she was passionate about through reduced-cost learning and shared her knowledge through online forums. It took courage and flexible thinking for Cass to find a different way to share her vocation as she accommodated the changes in her health status.

Whether it's fantasy or necessity, leaving our current work or vocation is something that many midlife women struggle with. There is bravery involved with any vocational choice, whether it is imagining a new path, taking steps on a new path, or remaining in the same place and accepting your current job and vocation for the foreseeable future.

What I admire most about women is that they are pragmatic; they have the wisdom and intuition to know what they need to do for themselves and those around them to thrive, and they are not afraid to do what must be done. In our vocation, sometimes we must be flexible and creative about the balance between what pays the bills and how we get our personal needs met. Though this isn't a new conundrum, it feels new to us because we may not have encountered this type of job dissatisfaction, unhappiness, or boredom before.

CONCLUSION

As I said before, this was a very challenging chapter to write, and it forced me to take another look at my own vocational choices, positive steps, and missteps I've made along the way. I leave you with several exercises and reflections that you can use to help guide your path in thinking about your own vocational life and how you can refine it for this stage of your life. Your vocational path is your own, and taking time to rethink your journey and make tweaks or to keep it the same is an important exercise at various points along the way. Because we are in midlife and have the benefit of perspective, I also believe that looking at how central (or not) your work life is can be an important part of introspection. It is my utmost hope that this chapter, the exercises, and the reflections allow you to move toward the best vocational life that you can create for this stage of your life.

VOCATIONAL SATISFACTION EXERCISE

Using figure 8.3, rate your overall vocational satisfaction on a scale from one to ten. There are several things to consider when rating your overall satisfaction, including *working conditions, colleagues, workload, autonomy, education and growth opportunities, variety of tasks, and the fit between you and the work environment.*

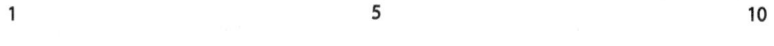

Figure 8.3. Vocational Satisfaction Scale

After you've determined your number, take a moment to define what that number means to you. How does the number reflect your satisfaction and dissatisfaction with your vocational life? (You can be both satisfied and dissatisfied with the same work—we are complex creatures.)

What values do you hold about your vocation and work?
How is your current job and/or vocation allowing you to live within your values (remember that your job and vocation can be different)?
How is your current job and/or occupation not aligning with your values?

Now, on a scale from one to ten, rate how burnout may impact your vocational experience using figure 8.4. Dimensions or constructs that are related to burnout include exhaustion, being overextended at work, cynicism, disengagement, and feeling ineffective. Signs that may indicate that you are not experiencing burnout can include feeling engaged in your work and having high levels of professional efficacy. (Note that these constructs are further defined by research from the Maslach Burnout Inventory.)

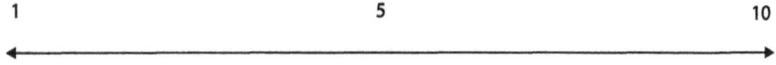

Figure 8.4. Burnout Scale

After you've determined your number, take a moment to define what that number means to you. How does the number reflect your level of burnout? *Note that burnout is a serious condition, and I encourage you to seek mental health treatment if you believe that you are experiencing high and/or debilitating levels of it.*

ADDITIONAL REFLECTION QUESTIONS

- How can you make your job work for you?
- How can you reframe one of the issues that you are experiencing at work to look at it differently?
- If you are experiencing heightened levels of job fatigue or burnout, what is one boundary you need to engage in to decentralize your work life from the rest of your life?

If you were to redraw your work-life balance pie chart to reflect how you want your life to look, how would it change?

Figure 8.5. Your Revised Work-Life Balance Pie Chart

What three steps will help recalibrate your pie chart from figure 8.2 to figure 8.5?

1. _____
2. _____
3. _____

FINAL REFLECTIONS

- What do you need to bring into the world that brings meaning to you?
- What about your vocation brings you joy or sense of purpose?
- Do you feel your vocation is still suitable for whom you are today?
- Are you still suitable for your vocation?
- Is your vocation giving you meaning?
- If not, do you quit or find other ways to bring meaning into what you do with your life?

BOOK RESOURCE LIST

(AKA my favorite books about work and vocational life balance.)

- *Designing Your New Work Life: How to Thrive and Change and Find Happiness and a New Freedom at Work* by Bill Burnett and Dave Evans (Vintage, 2021).
- *Getting' (Un)busy: Five Steps to Kill Busyness and Live with Purpose, Productivity, and Peace*, by Garland Vance (Author Academy Elite, 2019).
- *The No Club: Putting a Stop to Women's Dead-End Work*, by Linda Babcock, Brenda Peyser, Lise Vesterlund, and Laurie R. Weingart (Simon & Schuster, 2022).
- *The Book of Boundaries: Set the Limits That Will Set You Free*, by Melissa Urban (Dial Press, 2022).

CHAPTER NINE

LEISURE

When I was a little girl, my parents started taking me skiing. When I was two, they took me skiing without much success, other than me falling down a lot and freezing my hands in the snow. When I was about seven, they took me skiing again, but this time I was old enough to take lessons and learn some of the techniques that took me from falling to flying down the slopes. Oh, my word—freedom! If you've never been skiing, similar experiences might be coasting your bike down a hill, riding a roller coaster, or flying down the road with the top down on a convertible.

I grew up in the South, so my opportunities were few and far between, but my parents and I occasionally traveled for a few days of skiing or took day trips to resorts closer to our home. Although both of my parents were pretty good skiers, my dad was a natural athlete and, having been born in Germany, had access to skiing throughout his life. When he and my mother met, one of the things that they enjoyed doing was traveling to different spots in the northern United States and Canada for big trips. Since it was something that they valued, they shared their love of the sport with their kids, first with my sisters and later with me when I came along.

Skiing then is likely not how it is today (sadly, I haven't been skiing in years); back then, it was very much old equipment, buy your lift ticket, keep the same snow gear for as long as you can wear it (or get hand me downs), and pack your lunch to bring to the lodge to eat during the day. We were not après ski people; we were people who wanted to be out on the slopes enjoying good runs, challenging ourselves, and embracing the cold. The values that my parents passed down to me through skiing were to challenge myself both physically and mentally, to enjoy (relatively) low-cost, fun activities, and to create memories with the people I love.

One of my favorite memories is from my late high school/early college days when my dad and I went on a day trip to a ski resort. I was a novice at parallel skiing, but my dad was good. He coached me on my technique and followed me down the slopes, shouting out encouragement and tips to help improve my form. I can hear him now: "lean forward!" As the day went on, I got better and we were able to go down slopes faster and with greater ease, trying out black diamond runs. Always me in front and my dad behind, we loved speed and improving technique. One of my favorite memories of that day is seeing him in my peripheral vision; if I skied the slope down the left, he sliced right, and vice versa, so that we created a crisscross pattern in the snow. That day went on forever; that day was way too short. We did so many runs we almost forgot to stop and eat lunch; we were much later getting our gear off and heading home than we intended. I don't think we got home until 2:00 a.m., but what a day! That memory and others of skiing with my family are ones that I hold up as the hallmarks of true leisure; doing something in your free time because you enjoy it, something that is worth doing because it is so much fun. Taking this idea a step further, leisure can be activities that put you in a state of flow, which is a place of cognitive immersion, where you are so present, engrossed, and focused that time feels suspended.

I don't know about you, but the time that I set aside for leisure is far less than it was when I was younger. Even as I write this, I can feel the wellspring of joy and happy memories from skiing and other activities that I engage in for my enjoyment. And that's the goal of this chapter: to remind us that the joy and benefits of leisure are so important that we shouldn't leave them behind. As a midlife woman, so much of my life is about to-do lists and duties, which often causes me to shove my leisure activities into the background. I think about those lists and obligations often in relation to what some people call "deathbed regrets." These are the regrets we experience at the end of our lives; a well-documented one is "I wish I'd worked less and enjoyed my life more." When we're in our lives, particularly in the middle of our lives, we can feel pulled to meet the needs of many others—our children, partners, parents, friends, employers. Although these pulls are loud and important, if we don't take moments to stop, to explore what we do for fun, and to experience a sense of play in our lives, we are vulnerable to losing touch with our essence. In this chapter, we look at leisure and the role that it can play in our lives. We also examine how play and leisure can evolve throughout our lives and explore ways that we can incorporate them so that we can enjoy the benefit of a life fully lived.

WHAT LEISURE IS

As I began researching this chapter, I was struck by the limited research on the topics of leisure and midlife women. It became so challenging that I asked for help from one of my university's research librarians to help me find articles. Virginia, who is always game to help, said, "As a midlife woman, I take special interest in this search." Sadly, Virginia and I didn't have much luck. We found some interesting articles that inform this chapter, but as she wrote me in an email, "I have not found a ringer, that one great article that really brings midlife women's leisure experiences to the here and now." Without a "ringer" article, it's up to us to bring midlife women's leisure into the fore.

Leisure is freedom from work or duties; going a step beyond this, it is an activity that is absorbing, which gives you joy or fulfillment (hopefully both). In a world where there are many things we "have" to do, this is something that you *want* to do. In my experience (both personally and working with other women), barriers to engaging in leisure activities can include feeling guilty about doing something that isn't task-oriented and feeling selfish for wanting something of one's own. These activities can include physical activities like exercising or sports and creative activities such as painting or writing.

In an article about midlife leisure that I did find, the researcher noted that although midlife is a time of stressful events and life changes, many adults surveyed reported that they felt that it was the point in their lives at which they finally had time to find out who they were and explore their interests (Arnett, 2018). What the author highlighted was a midlife adult's search for eudaemonic well-being or, in more approachable language, an individual's search for existential purpose and well-being. One of the most salient ways to find one's existential purpose and well-being is to engage in leisure activities. These bring us closer to aspects of ourselves that are driven by our interests and desires, rather than by the demands of others.

When we engage in activities based on our leisure instincts, we may experience an increased sense of purpose and meaning. A sense of meaning can also promote our commitment to these tasks. When you experience the intrinsic value of something, you tend to want to repeat the activity. For example, imagine a toddler engaged in a game of peek-a-boo who doesn't want to stop playing. When our purpose, meaning, and commitment are united, we tend to report higher levels of positive physical and psychological health, as well as higher levels of overall life satisfaction (Holahan et al., 2011). While engaging in leisure activities, such as painting, we may find intrinsic satisfaction in experimenting, creating, and playing in a way that gives us purpose and meaning to express ourselves in a new way. The joy of painting and the personal satisfaction that it brings can be the reward that keeps us committed to the activity.

WHAT LEISURE ISN'T

I make a case for leisure and play in this chapter, but I want to have a brief discussion about what leisure *isn't*. I discuss joy, play, flow, and other important aspects that constitute leisure in upcoming sections. I even touch on some sneaky ways that leisure time can be hijacked: by getting through to-do lists, helping to care for others, and doing activities that others enjoy but that you do not. Leisure is more than a distraction; it isn't zoning out to social media or going through the motions of a craft activity because it's what your social group chose to do. Don't get me wrong, sometimes we do these things because it is what we need at the time, but that's not leisure. Think about a fun and leisure activity that gives you a sense of joy and rejuvenation. It feels so different than the so-so feeling you get from doing things that are not as invigorating (I'm talking to you, *Gilmore Girls* marathon). There is room for both leisure and zone-out time in our lives; knowing the benefits and consequences of our choices is important.

LEISURE AND PLAY

Engaging in activities for the sole pleasure of doing so is important for us now and for our future selves. When we consider the notion of eudaemonic well-being—the ongoing search for existential meaning and well-being—perhaps we need to harken back to our earlier lives and remember the role of play. Play, as defined by Brown (2009) "is an absorbing, apparently purposeless activity that provides enjoyment and a suspension of self-consciousness and a sense of time that is self-motivating" (p. 60). Many of our chosen leisure activities are based on play; however, to call it "play" in adulthood may carry stigma. My cousin and I chatted about this recently while discussing our never-ending to-do lists and the feeling that life keeps speeding up rather than slowing down. As children, we didn't have the duties that we do now, and play was expected of us. We had the time, freedom, and resources to engage in this important activity. When we are developing in infancy through adolescence, play serves multiple purposes: it allows us to problem-solve and try new things, it allows us to socialize with others or create solitary worlds, and it allows us to take risks in low-stakes ways.

As we grow into adulthood, our play habits can diminish over time. When my cousin and I looked at the cost versus benefit of play compared to completing our to-do lists, it felt as if getting tasks done was more important than playing. However, being task-oriented and forsaking play through leisure can have long-term consequences. Without playing through leisure activities, we risk becoming more fixed and rigid in our behaviors. We can lose interest in trying new things, become less curious about the world, and find less pleasure in our everyday lives. What science tells us is that those who play games, solve puzzles, and continue learning throughout their lives will enjoy fewer physical and cognitive declines later in life. Individuals who are regularly engaged in play and leisure activities tend to enjoy an overall better quality of life throughout the lifespan, with better mental and physical outcomes than their nonplaying peers. We need to make deposits in the "play bank" with leisure activities throughout our lives, not just in our childhood. If you read this and think, "What if I've permanently lost my sense of play?" don't panic. Your play drive is hardwired into your brain, just like your hunger drive; you can ignite it and get back in touch with it, but you do have to practice.

One way that you can explore your play and leisure interests is to identify your play personalities, as defined by Brown (2009, pp. 66–70). Note that there are eight personality types, and you won't necessarily fit into all of them, but you may find that you gravitate toward a few. Consider the ones that resonate with you and how they may fit into different parts of your life. You may be surprised. I remember having a session with my counselor after reading these. I explained that directing and organizing were fun for me and that may be part of the reason that I worked so much on those parts of my job—because they were the ones that felt like play. This was a mind-blowing revelation to me. In the previous chapter, we discussed how there can be parts of our work that we really enjoy, so keep in mind that these may be places in which our play drive is activated and we don't realize it. That said, the eight play personalities as defined by Brown (2009) are as follows.

- *Joker:* the personality type that is driven by nonsense, fun, jokes, and practical jokes. They may be driven to make people laugh, which can be a social strategy to gain acceptance.
- *Kinesthetic:* the personality type that is driven by the need to move. These individuals may be athletes but can include others who move to think. Their motivation is mostly based on wanting to engage in physical movement.
- *Explorer:* the personality type that is driven to see the world around them either literally or figuratively. These can be individuals who wish to see new places or who explore their world by interacting with new ideas or concepts.
- *Competitor:* the personality type that is driven to play games and wants to win. They experience a high from strategizing and achieving and tend to be individuals who believe that fun comes from being number one and tend to keep score to see where they land among the rest of the pack.
- *Director:* the personality type that is driven to plan and create events. They enjoy organizing and the power that comes from

being in charge. They tend to be the ones who can orchestrate events in which everything falls into place.
- *Collector:* the personality type that is driven by hunting and securing the most interesting objects or experiences. They tend to find joy in searching, either alone or with others, and procuring what they consider to be the best of their interests.
- *Artist/creator:* the personality type that is driven to create and make things. They tend to find joy in creating something that may be beautiful, functional, or perhaps both. These activities can be from scratch (such as making a hat out of yarn) or creation through objects (such as interior design).
- *Storyteller:* the personality type that is driven to create stories from their imagination. They tend to experience a high level of empathy and can intuit the motivations and emotions of the characters, which they describe masterfully.

MIDLIFE LEISURE

My friend and colleague, Leslie Stewart, holds a degree in leisure studies and is a certified recreational therapist. As I wrote this chapter, I thought that asking an expert to reflect on her leisure experiences may give some good insights into how we as midlife women can incorporate this important, and often neglected, part of our development into our lives. Leslie credited her early childhood and family experiences with helping her to develop into who she is: "I want as much joy as I can find and create. Life is hard and it doesn't get easier. Through my interests and hobbies, I found ways to do what I like and express myself fully." Leslie recalled that her mother would tell her and her siblings that if they were bored, they didn't have any imagination. As we discussed this further, Leslie reflected that part of this could have been that as a busy young mother of six, Joanne, her mom, didn't have time to entertain her children, and they had to learn to play on their own. It also turned into an excellent way for Leslie's parents to help each of their children foster their sense of individuality. Each of her siblings was interested in different types of play, and these play personalities have evolved into different leisure activities into adulthood.

Leslie identified a common thread throughout her play and leisure life, which was kinesthetics. As a young child, she was always moving, and this love of movement continued into her adulthood as she engaged in fitness through swimming and other physical activities. She recounted that one of the important ways she incorporated a sense of play and leisure into her life was by becoming a water safety instructor and later through her work as a certified recreational therapist and a physical therapist assistant. However, in midlife, several events and setbacks caused her to experience severe depression. While managing these difficult changes, she realized that she needed something that would help her to care for herself in other ways besides her physical activities. This is when she discovered her interest and love for art and creation.

"Finding things that I enjoyed doing, were inexpensive, and low risk became important for me at that point in my life. Being able to practice art opened a lot of opportunities for me to explore." Her early experiences in drawing classes led her to painting and weaving, all of which she does today. "I am still physically active; I really love inline skating. But being able to express myself through art, it was a paradigm shift of who and what I am and how I identify myself." She recalled another woman who referred to herself as an artist, which Leslie believed was so brave. Leslie now identifies herself as an artist. "Ultimately, I think of myself as a person who does, and I try to do what I like. This gives me a sense of fulfillment that is uniquely my own." From her education and experience, Leslie knows that finding new ways to enjoy leisure in midlife can be challenging. However, fostering a stronger sense of self, a better quality of life, and taking the opportunity to unlock her untapped potential are all reasons that Leslie is an advocate for midlife women's play and leisure time.

Lessons that I think are helpful for us from Leslie's experiences and training include the knowledge that there are always opportunities in life to explore new play and leisure experiences. Our early recollections about play can have lasting effects on how we see it in our lives now, so paying attention to those messages and what they tell us can be important. We may find that the negative or positive messages about play impact how we engage in leisure activities now. Some of our play drives may be with us our whole lives, like Leslie's desire for exercise and movement, or they may be part of our lives for certain seasons, like her midlife interest in art and creation. Exploration and flexibility can help us maintain our play drive. Finally, leisure activities can play an important role in helping us to cope when our lives become challenging. Like Leslie, we may find that during hard times our engagement in things that we're passionate or curious about, which give us joy, are the very things that we need most to cope. We also need to engage in leisure and play activities that give us a sense of fulfillment. In the next section, consider your narrative around leisure and play and the messages that you carry from your early life that inform your current ideas. What does your past tell you about leisure life now? How might it help you to create a new path for today and into the future?

CREATING A BRIDGE BETWEEN PLAY AND LEISURE

We all need to engage in leisure, play, and activities that give us a sense of fulfillment. Now that you have a better understanding of the play personalities, let's look at an exercise that can help you identify what your play preferences were in earlier life and how these (or others) may be expressed through your leisure activities during midlife. We're going to complete a play and leisure timeline to help you get started. I'll give you an example of how I completed this exercise (figure 9.1) and then a template that you can use for your own (figure 9.2).

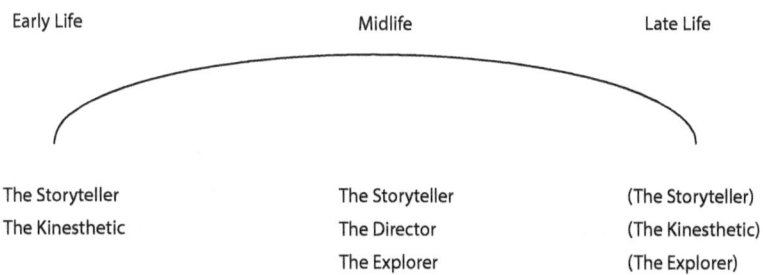

Figure 9.1. Sample Leisure Timeline

Now it's your turn. In the blank timeline arc (figure 9.2), write down the play languages that you engaged in during your early life and midlife. Use parentheses to indicate play personalities that you wish to explore now or in your future later life. You can include as many or as few play personality languages as you wish. I stopped at three, but you should write as many that makes sense for you.

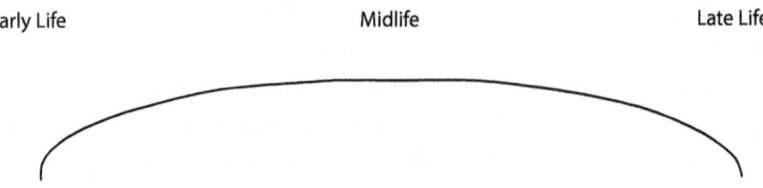

Figure 9.2. Your Leisure Timeline

REFLECTION

Next, consider your narrative around leisure and play and what messages you carry from your early life that inform your current ideas. What does your past tell you about leisure life now? How might it help you to create a new path for today and into the future? Think about not only your play personality, but how play is expressed in your life. The way you express play through your leisure activities changes over time. It's important to notice the difference between what feels like play and leisure, which can be the same thing, but aren't necessarily interchangeable. This is very much about how you feel when you're engaged in the activity.

Again, I provide some examples from my timeline that may be helpful.

Sample Leisure and Play Reflection
- Early Life Play Personalities and Expression: In my early life, my main play languages were storyteller and kinesthetic. I loved being read to, learning to read on my own, and creating narratives for my playthings. I was also active in dancing, skiing, bike riding, and playing with my dog. Many of my activities were more solitary, some by circumstances and some by my choice given my temperament.
- Midlife Play Personalities and Expression: In midlife, I have kept my storyteller play language; I am a voracious reader, and I am fascinated

by my work with students and clients and how the stories of their lives influence how they are as people. I have grown into my director play language through my personal life and work; I love executing a project and seeing things come together from beginning to end. Finally, I am a true explorer, again with my students and clients, but also deeply interested in traveling to new places to understand how others live.
- Late Life Play Personalities and Expression Wishes: Although I am not in late life, I imagine that storyteller play language will remain with me. As I imagine a life that may be less busy with responsibilities, play languages I would like to explore include getting back in touch with my kinesthetic play language and continuing my play language of explorer.
- The differences and similarities between play and leisure: For me, the best way to notice the difference between when something feels like play and leisure or leisure alone is my absorption level. For example, when I am reading a good book that I just can't put down, I will ignore everything else so I can stay in the story. This feels like playing to me. However, when engaged in a physical activity like weightlifting, I do it as a leisure activity; it feels good to my body, but I don't have that same sense of absorption or joy as I do when I've found a great story. Exercise feels good, and it is leisurely, but it isn't play.
- Midlife Reflection on Leisure: Because so much of my life feels like "duties" right now, I notice that I find play in the things that I am required to do, rather than engaging in any additional things for leisure or play. For example, I engage in my director play language when I coordinate programs for my job. Although it doesn't provide the same level of joy and absorption as true play or leisure, I realize that there is more leisure in my life than I recognized when I see this part of my life through a play and leisure lens; it also makes me realize that my definition of leisure at this stage of my life needs to be flexible.

Your Leisure and Play Reflection
- Early Life Play Personalities and Expression
- Midlife Play Personalities and Expression
- Late Life Play Personalities and Expression Wishes
- The Differences and Similarities between Play and Leisure
- Midlife Reflection on Leisure

BARRIERS TO LEISURE

Here's what's challenging about leisure: we know the reasons why it's good for us and the reasons why we can't seem to find the time for it. What research shows is that during the last forty years, women consistently have less quality time to devote to leisure activities than men. In one article, this quote stood out: "Leisure research indicates that women have less personal time and receive less private space, fewer resources, and less tolerance and respect than their male partners for pursuing the activities, especially the leisure activities they enjoy and find fulfilling" (Stalp, Radina, & Lynch, 2008). The idea that *partnered* women have less time for leisure is supported more recently in a Pew Research Center report from 2013 (Parker &Wang, 2013).

In addition to having less time to engage in leisure, barriers to women engaging in physical leisure activities can include fatigue, health problems, and safety concerns (Hall, 2007). As we grow older and have more responsibilities, we may find that our stamina decreases over time. These issues coupled with health constraints can make engaging in physical activities less appealing. For example, in my own life, I've had to take a medication with side effects that include dizziness and fatigue. While I was on the medication, certain physical activities weren't available to me, like hiking or yoga inversions, because I wasn't able to sustain these activities for long. Limitations can feel demoralizing and sometimes the consequences are feeling angry or depressed and withdrawing or quitting activities that previously gave you joy. It should also be mentioned that hormonal changes that occur in midlife, such as menopause, can also result in fatigue, which can impact women's capacity to engage in certain activities as well.

Resources are also major barriers that stop many women from being able to engage in leisure. When I refer to "resources," I am talking about money, time, and opportunity. Many women with whom I work say that if it comes between doing something for themselves or giving their children opportunities, like enrolling them in dance class, they put their resources toward their children. This is a value that resonates with many of us. Although it is important to give opportunities to our loved ones, we also need to be able to measure the cost if we don't invest some resources into ourselves. The question becomes, if I were to funnel some resources into myself (time, money, opportunity), what might that look like? I hear many women say that they enjoy helping to take care of others, and it is true that there is a high level of satisfaction in caretaking your kids, grandkids, parents, and partner, but this isn't leisure and being honest with yourself about that is important.

Another issue that comes up for many women is safety and leisure, which is typically linked to activities that happen outside the home. Many women identify with not feeling safe engaging in certain activities alone, such as running, which can be a major barrier to accessing leisure. Unfortunately, the world is not always a safe place for women. Acknowledging that the consequences of this means curtailing certain activities is a sad reality for many. This can include more than physical activities. For example, my friend Sarah is an excellent potter, and the pottery co-op that she once used was located in an isolated part of town. If she was there working alone, she took very specific precautions to ensure that she felt safe and secure in the building. To her, the benefits of engaging in her art outweighed the fear that she had for personal safety, and she took care to make certain that she was as safe as she could be. What makes me sad about this example, and many others, is that women must think about their own safety in ways that many of our male counterparts never do.

A final barrier we discuss here is what to do when your leisure activities seem to be lost to you. What I mean is when the things that you used to enjoy are no longer interesting to you or you can't do them anymore because of a particular barrier (cost, opportunity, physical, or emotional constraints). When this happens, it can be so hard because you're casting about for something to help reignite a spark and nothing seems to work. Like Leslie's story, sometimes becoming curious and trying new things can be a way to engage, by trial and error, in finding a passion. Here's the thing: when we're exploring new activities, we can try them out but not necessarily commit. Though that sounds like fun, it can be frustrating to try many things and feel as though nothing fits. This is when noticing the difference in how you feel when you are trying a new activity becomes important. If you find something fun, absorbing, and interesting, it may be something worth trying again. My friend Mimi tried many things before she got into kayaking. She loves it because it allows her to see the world from waterways; navigating through rapids engages her problem-solving skills, and getting into nature gives her a sense of peace that she doesn't find in other places. Conversely, my sister has continued to struggle to find activities that she considers leisure. I think this is because she, like me, is hardwired to get her to-do list done and less apt to give in to her play drive. Among her, our cousin, and me, you can see that the women in our family have issues with leisure and play! You may be like us, and if so, don't lose hope. According to Brown (2009), one of the best ways to ignite the play drive is to start with movement. This might be putting on some favorite music and bopping in your car; it could be playing with water guns; it could be taking a walk. Whatever gets you moving, do it, and then start to notice your instincts and play drive when they kick in. You may feel a sense of calm, a small smile on your face, an easing in your mind. These are the clues that leisure and play are closer than you think.

NO SPECIFIC PRESCRIPTION FOR LEISURE

I would love to be able to give us all a set prescription for leisure that denotes the parameters for how it should look in your life. What we know is that leisure contributes to well-being and that it is unique to the individual. There are overall brain benefits, social benefits, and physical benefits to play and leisure, but what works for one doesn't work for all. In an article about the benefits theory of leisure well-being, researchers discussed specific categories of leisure activities that meet individuals' needs. These categories include basic needs, growth needs, and satisfaction needs, based on individual personality traits (Sirgy, Uysal, & Kruger, 2017).

Women's basic needs in leisure may offer safety, health, economic, sensory, and escape benefits. Safety means that the activity is safe or that safety measures are taken to ensure that one will not get hurt, such as wearing a helmet when trail riding. Health benefits of an activity promote physical health, such as walking, stretching, or weightlifting. Economic benefits can be an activity's affordability or cost-effectiveness for the consumer. Sensory benefits include the experience of the activity or what follows, such as a massage or acupuncture session (and its aftereffects). Finally, "escape" allows the woman to suspend her daily activities and duties and enjoy being "away" by engaging in an activity that is not part of her normal routine.

Women's growth needs can include how leisure activities benefit them or are related to aesthetics, morality, mastery, relatedness, and distinctiveness. Leisure activities that benefit women's growth needs could include participating in a book club for women living in the same neighborhood. Aesthetics are related to the overall feel and experience of the activity, for example, visiting an art museum. Morality needs can be met by engaging in activities that benefit a particular group or charity organization, such as children's schools or a favorite nonprofit organization. Women's mastery needs can be achieved with activities that allow them to increase their knowledge, skills, or expertise in a particular area, similar to Leslie's growth as an artist. Relatedness means being involved in a leisure activity in which participants have common experiences and social interaction. It can be like the book club example mentioned earlier or something very different, like a group of ladies who explore national parks together. Finally, distinctiveness refers to leisure activities that allow women to carve out their unique way of being and showcase these for themselves and others.

Finally, leisure activities should relate to your personal preferences (and likely are) based on your unique personality traits. Knowing if you are more introverted or extroverted, if you like activities that are organized or free flowing, and if you are drawn to physical activity or sensory experiences all help you to narrow down the types of activities you enjoy and the needs you are trying to fulfill through leisure. As you continue to refine what you want to do (or not do) for fun, it's important to remember that your way of playing is unique to you. Although you may engage in certain activities to bond with others (such as camping because it is what your partners or friends enjoy) and they may be fun, they may not be as fulfilling as the activities that you do which are truly meaningful to you. Leisure is a place where only you can say what you like, without the influence of others. Which makes leisure wholly unique and sometimes challenging.

MAKING A LEISURE PLAN EXERCISE

Our time spent playing and engaging in leisure hinges on our ability to make it a priority. The resources that we need to have a healthy leisure life include money, time, and opportunity. As I wrote this chapter, the thought that kept circling my head was, *I hope that readers get mad about all of the barriers and limitations that may come with their attempts at leisure and play, and this catalyzes them to find room for it in their lives.* A full life is a life with play and leisure, one in which women have the right to enjoy these pursuits just as much as our male counterparts. Although we are not always offered the same opportunities for this important pursuit, we must be empowered to take them when we can. The long-term ramifications of a life that includes leisure and play are healthier experiences in older age and a better quality of life.

Thinking back to your leisure timeline and your leisure and play reflection, complete the reflections below and plan for leisure. You deserve joy, play, flow, and time—now more than ever.

REFLECTION

- What are you doing for leisure, if anything?
- What benefits do you notice from this activity?
- Have any of the things you used to do for leisure turned into obligations? Do you need to change how you engage in these activities?
- How could you explore new leisure activities that you are curious about?
- What would stop you from exploring new activities?
- What could be a plan for minimizing those obstacles?

Sample Leisure Plan: *I will plan one leisure activity for myself within the next month using a SMART (specific, measurable, achievable, realistic, and timely) goal. Once the activity is completed, I'll commit to reflecting on my experience and noticing what I enjoyed and didn't enjoy about the activity.*

Sample SMART Leisure Goal:
- *I will go to the library next week to explore the travel section and check out books about nearby cities that I want to visit during the next year.*
- *I will sign up for an open mic night and complete a five-minute stand-up routine by the end of June.*

- *I will start training tomorrow for a 5K scheduled for September. I'll download a training app on my phone and sign up with friends so that it is social and so that I have accountability.*

Your SMART leisure goal: _____
_____
_____
_____
_____

Reflection after you've completed your goal: _____
_____
_____
_____
_____

CHAPTER TEN

BELIEF SYSTEMS AND SPIRITUAL HEALTH

Growing up in the South, religious doctrines and spirituality surrounded me from a very young age. My first foray into religion began when I started kindergarten at the same Catholic school that my father attended when he was a teen. Although my education there gave me a very strong foundation, it also left me very confused about religion. Imagine me, a little kindergartener, gathering with my class during circle time for our religion class taught by the school's religion teacher, Mrs. Clark, and our principal, Sister Amelia. These ladies were there to teach us our first lessons on what it meant to be part of a religion in ways that our young minds could understand.

But before we could get started, they needed to make something clear. Although all of the class would be taking religion classes together, not all of us would go through the same confirmation rituals at the end of third grade. Why, may you ask? Well, because some of us weren't members of the faith for various reasons. In my case, I wasn't "eligible" for Catholic baptism and confirmation because my mother had been divorced (*gasp!*), and I am the product of her second marriage. But not to worry: no matter if we were going through confirmation or not, God loved us all. Thus began my long and very confusing relationship with religion and spirituality.

I think the most profound lesson my young mind took from this experience was that even if there was a "God" who loved us all, there always would be a division between how people experienced the divine, with some being on one side of an invisible line and the rest of us on the other side. A big life lesson and insight for a five-year-old. I remember asking my parents for an explanation of my kindergarten experience, and they told me not to worry about it, that I should enjoy the stories and lessons and remember that the more important school lessons would be about learning my letters and numbers. I didn't grow up in a particularly religious household (as if you couldn't tell), and my parents attempted to instill in me a strong moral compass and lessons of right and wrong to guide my thoughts and behavior. I chalk this up to their negative experiences with religion and the great parental prerogative to do things differently than what had been done to them.

Fast-forward to my teenage and early adult years, when I began attending church services to better understand the religiosity that my friends discussed in carpool and because I was dating a boy whose family was religious. Let's just say that although I found the rituals interesting, these communities were not for me in the long term. When I was a young professional, I was introduced to a division of my counseling organization called the Association for Spiritual, Ethical, and Religious Values in Counseling (ASERVIC). Here I was a part of a group of seekers who identified differently: some were religious, whereas others were spiritual, and still others were agnostic or atheist. Yet we all came together to discuss the powerful dynamics that religion, spirituality, existentialism, and ethics played in our lives as humans and counselors.

I can't tell you what a relief it was to find a group of people who were open to individual differences in spiritual backgrounds, who didn't "other" based on religious affiliation or nonaffiliation, and who agreed that certain human rights are inalienable to all. What this group did for me was to rekindle my interest and curiosity in what religious, spiritual, and existential seeking can bring to my life. Although I still question how I can continue to develop as a spiritual person, what I know is that I am a more contented soul for knowing that it's okay to draw upon the principles of religion, spirituality, existentialism, and morality to guide my inner and outer life, regardless of whether I am a part of what is considered an "organized" group.

This chapter aims to explore and understand our place in the world as we move through midlife. Our connection to others, paths for healing from wounds, and the acceptance of challenges and changes in life can evolve as we get older. Our existential, spiritual, and religious beliefs can become a cornerstone for helping us to make meaning at this phase of life. Before we go further, it's important to define terms regarding spirituality, religion, agnosticism, atheism, and existentialism for this chapter. According to Merriam-Webster, *spiritual* is defined as something related to sacred matters, whereas *religion* is a personal set or institutionalized system of religious attitudes, beliefs, and practices. Note that the word *spiritual* is a bit less rigid than *religion*. *Agnostic* refers to one who is not committed to believing in either the existence *or* the nonexistence of God or a god. In contrast, an atheist is a person who does not believe in the existence of God or any gods. Finally, *existential* is defined as relating to or affirming existence. Regardless of where you belong on the spectrum of belief systems, you belong in this chapter. We all seek to find our place in the world, and belief systems serve as guiding principles for how we live our lives. However, these beliefs and the paths that individuals follow can vary from person to person.

Remember way back in chapter 7, when the basic tenets of harmonious disagreement were introduced? Our discussion centered on how we can engage and interact with individuals with whom we don't share the same values, and that we can respect that we each have the right to engage in our values. The irony is that the practice of harmonious disagreement evolved out of religious exchange—yet religious disagreement is the epicenter of so much of the conflict that our world has experienced in its history. I want you to consider how you can move through this chapter with an open mind and concentrate on how your values influence your experience of the world. This can be challenging because often there are groups of people who feel judged based on their religious beliefs or nonbelief. Where I live, there are many religious-based counselors, and clients come to me in shame or fear of identifying as agnostic or atheistic. This chapter isn't about creating judgment about different groups; it is about examining your belief system, where you lie on the spectrum of religion, spirituality, and existentialism, and how that impacts your sense of self. Note that as this chapter continues, I use "belief systems" to encompass spirituality, religion, agnosticism, atheism, and existentialism; this term is intended to be inclusive of all readers.

KNOWING YOUR STORY

Understanding and mining your own story and belief system history is an important part of knowing where you are now and how you may evolve in the future. An interesting way to examine this is to create an "I Am" poem. These poems are traditionally used to look at a wide variety of cultural identities, but in this case, we will adapt it to reflect on our own experiences and the development of our belief system. The exercise itself can be long or short; the only rules are that each sentence begins with "I am" and tells the story through the lens of your past, present, and future belief systems. I provide an abbreviated example of my "I am" poem and then it's your turn to reflect and create your own.

Before we get started, a word on spiritual and religious wounds and trauma. Many among us have experienced abuse and harm in spiritual and religious communities and in the name of specific religions. If these are issues that you are managing, it may be best to skip this exercise. These wounds are real, and they are important, but it is up to you to determine when and if you wish to work on them, preferably with professional support. This type of exercise can be emotional for individuals who don't readily identify as victims or survivors of spiritual or religious abuse, so go easy with your work through this chapter and pay attention to your reactions. Keep yourself safe as we move through.

"I AM" EXERCISE

My poem:

> I am a child of God, but not a child of your God; I don't belong in the same way that you belong. I am other.
>
> I am a seeker who looks to find a place when one was not offered to me; knowing my spiritual life is something that is just beyond my reach and without anyone to guide me.
>
> I am alone in my existential quest, and I know that I am never alone because of the universalizing truth that we are all together.

Now it's your turn. Your poem can be as long or as brief as you wish; it can be very specific or abstract in its descriptions. You may create distinct images that arise for you in your recollections or create a general sense of feelings. This is your unique work to explore your belief system.

Your poem:

_____
_____
_____
_____
_____
_____
_____

REFLECTION QUESTIONS

- What does your poem reveal to you about your spiritual life?
- Are there ways that your spiritual life has changed from past to present?
- Do you see an expression of stability or change in your description of your spiritual life from present to future?
- Are the values that you aligned with in chapter 2 reflected in any way through your poetry?

UNDERSTANDING BELIEF SYSTEM DEVELOPMENT AND ITS PLACE IN OUR LIVES

Belief systems serve an important role in our culture; they can provide a sense of connectedness to ourselves, others, and the universe. For those who are part of religious institutions, these communities can be opportunities to share space with like-minded individuals who mutually support and care for each other and are unified by the same beliefs and rituals. For others, a belief system path may be more individual and solitary. The purpose of these systems is to help us make meaning for ourselves and the world around us, particularly when so much of life is ambiguous and can feel illogical.

Belief systems can offer comfort, letting us know that we will be "okay" when our lives feel chaotic or uncertain; they also can allow us to marvel at the beauty of the everyday and celebrate the wonderful things that happen in our lives. Ultimately, our belief systems help us to determine our priorities, the values that we choose to live by, and offer a template for how we see ourselves in the world. These are measures that transcend the metrics we often use to define ourselves—our relationships or our work—and get to the core of who we truly are when we are alone and quiet in our heads. To harken back to our childhood, it's the version of Jiminy Cricket that lives within you; it's your true consciousness and conscience.

Our belief systems develop and are cultivated over time. What I mean is that there are noticeable maturation stages that happen throughout an individual's lifetime, in which they move from more simplistic to sophisticated ways of thinking about their belief systems and the world around them. Two of the most famous theories that help us conceptualize the development of belief systems are Kohlberg's stages of moral development and Fowler's stages of faith development. Though both theories have their strengths and drawbacks, they give a roadmap for thinking about beliefs.

Lawrence Kohlberg was the psychologist who built upon Jean Piaget's developmental work to devise the stages of moral development. These stages begin in early childhood and follow individuals throughout their lifespan. The stages that are most germane to adulthood are the ones associated with postconventional morality, which includes moral decisions that are based on social contract and universal ethics. In Kohlberg's *social contract stage*, individuals understand that our society is filled with others who have contrasting opinions and values that should be respected. People who have attained this developmental stage tend to understand that laws are flexible social contracts and laws that don't serve the common good should be changed to better align with societal needs. Specific behaviors or actions of folks in this stage of development may include advocating for changes to law and policy, such as changes to promote equity and individual rights. Those within the social contract stage also understand the validity of different perspectives and that compromise can be a path toward change that supports more of the common good.

Universal ethics, Kohlberg's final proposed stage, is one in which very few people achieve, he purported. Within universal ethics, individuals create their moral principles, which may deviate from societal laws. A quick note: not all societal laws are equitable; cast your mind back to chapter 1 and our discussion on women's suffrage, the right to vote, and barriers that still existed for minority women even after the nineteenth amendment was passed. Examples of principles that may underlie individuals' beliefs can include equity (valuing others no matter their background), dignity (belief in the inherent worth of all people), and respect (upholding the rights and beliefs of others). People at this stage are more likely to challenge laws or norms if they see them as harmful or unjust. Again, consider the suffragettes who protested for women's voting rights or the civil rights movement.

Another way to conceptualize belief system development is through James Fowler's Spiritual Development model, which examines at stages of faith and faith development. As with Kohlberg, Fowler took his cue from Piaget, developing a model that examines scaffolded spiritual development through stages over time. The three stages that pertain most to midlife spiritual development are the *individuative-reflective stage*, the *conjunctive stage*, and the *universalizing stage*. The individuative-reflective stage occurs in adulthood and is marked by the realization that belief systems are internalized and a growing awareness of the limitations that these systems may impose. Folks at this stage begin to question their beliefs, particularly when they begin to see contradictions between their belief systems and their experience of the world. An example of this might be a belief system in which all life matters, but certain groups of people are ostracized or excluded for some reason. This internalized questioning can cause discomfort, cognitive dissonance, and pain; for some, this stage results in the rejection of faith, and for others it can lead to a stronger conviction.

Fowler's next phase is called the conjunctive stage, which typically does not occur before midlife. At this stage, individuals begin to understand that some experiences and aspects of belief are not explained by the rational mind and will remain ambiguous. People at this stage of faith development are comfortable having conversations about faith with others and use these conversations to challenge themselves and revise their own beliefs and insights about their belief systems. The last phase in Fowler's model is the universalizing stage, in which individuals see all humanity as one and take self-sacrificing action to care for others. Very few individuals reach this developmental level; Mother Theresa is a popular archetype for this stage.

Both models are useful in conceptualizing belief system development, and both have their drawbacks. Stage development models imply a linear progression between stages, in which a person moves from one to the next, like checking boxes. This isn't so. Our development can be dependent upon our experiences, and our experiences vary as we grow. So although we may be highly developed in one area, we may be less developed in other areas of our lives. Therefore, we may move between stages during different parts of our lives as we continuously grow and develop. It should also be noted that these theorists were white men whose theories were based on other European white men. Because of this, we know that women and diverse individuals were often not at the forefront of theorists' minds. Finally, Fowler's model didn't delve into how these models apply to individuals who identify as agnostic or atheist. Despite these limitations, developmental models are a useful way to conceptualize belief systems so that we have a frame of reference to understand spiritual functioning.

RESEARCH ON BELIEF SYSTEMS AND HEALTH OUTCOMES

Much of the academic literature regarding the impact of religion and spirituality on overall well-being states that engaging in religious or spiritual practices offers positive health benefits compared to those who do not participate in these practices (agnostic, atheist, existentialist). It appears that the metaphorical card deck is stacked in favor of those with belief systems based on religiosity or spirituality. However, there are a lot of studies about the relative health benefits of religion and spirituality, but there are not many scientific studies that examine the same indicators for those who identify as nonreligious. Reasons for the gap in research include a lack of interest on the part of researchers, a general lack of funding for this type of research, and difficulty finding nonreligious comparison groups due to stigmatization.

Within academic literature, there is a great deal of support for the idea that those who hold belief systems that are religious or spiritual tend to have better health outcomes than those whose belief systems are nonreligious. Typical measures of health outcomes include physical indices (body mass index [BMI] and activities of daily living [ADL]) and psychological indices (social supports, positive psychological functioning) (Koenig, King, & Carson, 2012). Interestingly, there's been a recent push in academic literature for research into the overall health outcomes of individuals whose belief systems are nonreligious. The impetus for this may be the growing number of individuals who report no religious affiliation. In a Gallup poll completed in 2023, approximately 22 percent of survey respondents indicated that they did not identify with any religion and 28 percent of respondents indicated that religion and spirituality are not important to their daily lives (Gallup, 2023).

Regardless of belief system, what more recent literature tells us is that the perceived health disparities between those who hold religious or spiritual belief systems compared to those whose belief systems are nonreligious are not as clearly defined as was previously thought. In a 2016 study completed by Hayward and colleagues, researchers found that some whose belief systems were characterized as nonreligious tended to have better physical health indicators when compared to their religious counterparts. However, these same researchers found that those with religious and spiritual belief systems tended to have better psychological health outcomes than their nonreligious counterparts.

Women in midlife tend to identify their belief systems as spiritually, religiously, or nonreligiously affiliated; fewer women than men identify as atheistic or agnostic. Ultimately, it could be that our belief systems are largely influenced by our personality traits, with some of us being more inclined to spiritual and religious belief systems, whereas others are more inclined toward nonreligious/spiritual belief systems (Caldwell-Harris, 2012). But what is the "secret sauce" that belief communities have that can help buffer health outcomes? Some of the benefits include having a social support network, having a framework of psychological tools that assist in coping with adverse experiences, and promotion of self-control, which can lead to better health habits (Hayward et al., 2016).

Belonging to a community and having a social support network is likely one of the greatest benefits associated with religious or spiritual belief system affiliation. As discussed in chapter 7, midlife women experience many barriers to engaging in social connection, and the benefit of a belief system community is the built-in opportunity to engage with others. Additionally, the challenges that midlife women face at this life stage—such as caring for others, personal health concerns, and so forth—are systemic, extending beyond the individual. Having a community of people who can help "fill in" when women are stretched thin can be invaluable. This might include having affordable summer camps for kids or eldercare opportunities for ailing parents through a church community. For better or worse, there are fewer community-based, secular examples of these types of support systems in our current culture.

Having a framework of coping tools to help manage adverse experiences is another perceived strength of religious and spiritual communities. One of the premier researchers for religious coping is Ken Pargament, who has spent his professional life studying this subject and applying it to therapeutic practice. According to his research, religious coping can be broken down into two main types: positive and negative. Positive religious coping includes reframing challenges as positives or growth opportunities, seeing a higher power as a partner guiding one through challenges, and seeking a higher power's love and care (Pargament, 2011). Negative religious coping includes seeing challenges as a punishment from a higher power, passively depending on a higher power to solve one's problems, and coping with struggles alone and without a higher power's help (Pargament, 2011).

Finally, religious and spiritual belief communities often promote and encourage the practice of self-control within one's existence and in community with others. Examples of individual self-control can include religious communities' social contracts to limit the intake of intoxicants or certain foods. Community self-control might be illustrated in acts of service and personal sacrifice of the individual for the good of others. Having other individuals who are engaged in activities separately but together (and with a higher power) provides accountability, which can make behavior maintenance or changes easier to manage.

Although these three benefits are seen as the main reasons that individuals engaged in religious and spiritual communities may have better health outcomes than their nonreligious counterparts, it doesn't mean that these benefits don't exist outside of religious and spiritual communities or that nonreligious people don't have opportunities to engage in these benefits in a secular way. As I stated earlier, there is very limited research on the experiences of nonreligious people and their overall health outcomes. However, a community can be built in less formal ways and through secular means by joining clubs and social friendship circles. Given the decline in attendance and membership in organized religious and spiritual communities, secular organizations are likely to fill this need for many in a more desirable way. Because the inherent benefits of religious and spiritual organizations are well documented in academic literature but not in secular ones, it is unclear if secular support systems offer the same protective health factors. Ultimately, the perception of support and benefits is up to the individual engaged in the group. Meaning is one of the most important paradigms that our belief systems offer us, and in the next section, I discuss how meaning-making is an imperative part of our midlife journey.

BELIEF SYSTEMS AND MEANING

When I was around fourteen, I was a candy striper at a local hospital. (I believe the new term is a "junior volunteer.") I won't go into the vagaries of how this was an early education of free emotional labor, women's indoctrination into the ethic of care, or an opportunity to exploit the good intentions of a young person. In retrospect, it was likely all those things, and it was also an opportunity to give back to my community, learn about medical care, and explore career paths. What I could never have known was that on my first day as a volunteer, I had an experience of helping that has stayed with me for my entire life and became the basis of my career as a counselor.

My supervising administrator took me to the pediatrics unit, where I was pointed to the room of an infant, probably about ten months old, who was alone. The other children in the unit had someone, a parent or other caregiver, tending to them and keeping them company. This little boy was so small and thin. I wondered if he was on his own most of the time; maybe he had busy parents, or maybe he didn't have anyone who cared for him. I don't know. He was crying and despondent, and as I tried to engage with him, I will never forget the look in his eyes. He was so young and old all at once; his eyes were watchful and wary. I think that he had experienced a lot already in his young life and wasn't ready to trust anyone. My training now tells me that this infant had suffered, but at that time all I knew was that I wanted to help this small soul and the skill to do so was beyond my reach.

I wish I had a happy ending to his story, but I don't have any ending, because I went on with my life and he with his. I believe the reason that his face and the look in his eyes have stayed with me is that it was the first time I truly could recognize wounds in others and recognized my inability to help. And although I've become very perceptive in finding the wounds in others and helping them heal, I still struggle to recognize my own. How many times do you look in the mirror and truly recognize your wounds? We see them in others but often fail to look at the vulnerability within ourselves. Our belief systems offer us a way to make meaning in our lives, to hold our vulnerability as precious, and to aid us in healing wounds. What other ways can our belief systems help us navigate our lives?

Our belief systems offer us a way to relate to the world and others in a healthy way; they also provide us with a blueprint for how we understand our normal life development. Our belief systems help us to find a path to transcend hardships and develop resilience in the face of adversity. As midlife women, we've managed hardships in our past and will have more in the second half of our lives. How has navigating hardships helped you to develop a better understanding of what you believe about yourself and the world? What tools have you used to help cope with life's challenges? These answers are individual and specific, but they can tell you a lot about how your belief system influences your worldview.

Our belief systems also offer us a way to understand our values and how we want to be in the world. Consider the value sort you completed at the very beginning of this book; it had everything to do with your internalized belief systems! Perhaps some of your choices didn't surprise you, but perhaps some did, and these surprises might be indicative of your life's evolution. Speaking in terms of values is helpful because it is a way to be inclusive of all religions, faiths, belief systems, and philosophies. It is important to be inclusive because our values and the meaning that we assign to ourselves and others are universal experiences that all people must navigate in this life; these experiences are not exclusive to people in one tradition or another.

Another way that our belief systems offer us a framework for life is by providing us a way to navigate the wounds that we experience in the world; yet those life wounds can become the catalyst that causes us to question whether these beliefs still serve us. In more extreme cases, life wounds can result in ruptures or complete breaks from our previously held beliefs. When this happens, we can find ourselves adrift, confused, angry, and scared. In the next section, we look at how our spiritual wounds can impact us and how we relate to ourselves and others in the world. Understanding these wounds can help us navigate disruptions in our belief systems and help us reformulate our worldview in ways that make sense after difficult experiences.

UNDERSTANDING OUR WOUNDS

Just as much as our happy and nurturing experiences help to shape how we see the world, our challenges, traumas, and existential wounds are just as important in forming our worldview. Wounds, or traumas, can vary depending upon the person, and what is traumatic for me may not be the same thing that is traumatic for you. In psychotherapy parlance, there are two types of traumas: "big T" and "little t." A "big T" trauma is something that most of us would think of as traumatic, such as living through a natural disaster or witnessing or being a victim of a violent act. A "little t" trauma is smaller and more personally dependent, such as experiencing bullying and microaggressions in our social interactions. Traumas and wounds can have a cumulative effect on us, meaning that if you experience a lot of them in quick succession, you may find yourself less resilient over time.

How do we know when we're wounded? Oftentimes we feel battered, and that feeling washes through us in our bodies, minds, and spirits. When I work with clients, some of them can pinpoint exactly where their wounds originate; some have a harder time uncovering the origin story of their wounds. The easiest wounds to identify include those that were caused externally, such as aggressions inflicted on us by other people or systems. The more insidious wounds are those that fester internally, which perhaps started as an external wound that we internalized and changed the narrative of how we feel about ourselves and how we see the world around us.

A former client who experienced the end of her marriage provides an example of this. When she uncovered new information about her relationship with her spouse, the image that she had of her life and the life she had built with her former husband was shattered. Although the end of a marriage is traumatic, it wasn't just the "big T" trauma of the end of the relationship that felled this woman, it was also the "little t" traumas of a community that was not supportive of the divorce. Once this client believed that she had the support of her community, including her faith community, for difficult times, but she was left feeling as though she was not supported. Not only had the client lost her marital relationship and the love and security she believed was part of the relationship, but she also lost her faith community in an equally devastating manner.

Not all wounds are directly related to our faith communities, but when they are, it can feel like a double betrayal: a rejection from both one's community and one's higher power. My client had to take a step back from her belief system and her faith community to make sense of these wounds and reformulate how to move forward with an altered worldview. After examination, her core values hadn't changed, but her relationship with that faith community and her ability to maintain trust with the people within it was forever different. In some ways, the rupture with that faith community was irreparable.

Part of this client's story—and all our journeys when navigating wounds—is forgiveness. Our belief systems provide us with an understanding of how we can forgive ourselves and others in the face of transgressions of trust. I say "transgressions of trust" because I believe that these are the seminal wounds that we experience. We give our trust to someone or something, and it is violated. When we experience violations of trust, we engage in forgiveness so that we can first trust ourselves again. Then we can let go of the wounds that others have caused and (perhaps) build trust with them as well. However, we must be aware that forgiveness of ourselves doesn't mean that we are compelled to forgive others if it isn't healthy for us to do so. There are large transgressions for which no forgiveness can be given and to say that one "must" forgive can cause additional trauma to a victim or survivor.

For my client, the primary work of healing her wounds was her forgiveness work. She felt "stuck": if she had been a different person, if she had been a better religious devotee, or if she had paid more attention, she would not have been wounded and betrayed in the ways that she was. This was her crucible; she had never experienced a situation in which she had to forgive herself for being human and for trusting people she believed had her best interests at heart. These are not the wounds we had as children when we skinned our knees from falling off our bikes; these are the psychic injuries that change our perceptions of ourselves. Her work is ongoing, and it was the catalyst for finding a new faith community and new metrics for measuring how she could trust others in the future.

As we think about our wounds as midlife women, we can look back on the challenges we've navigated and find solutions that can work for us to move forward. We are capable of self-healing for the simple reason that some wounds heal on their own by necessity. Questions to ask yourself when tending to your wounds can include:

- What does my belief system tell me about admitting that I am wounded?
- How can I ask for help with wounds and traumas that I need help to understand?
- How does this wound influence my beliefs about myself and how I see the world?
- If this wound may never fully heal, how can I learn to live with it, despite it?
- How can I work to forgive in relation to this wound?
- How can I work to trust in relation to this wound?

OUR BELIEF SYSTEMS ARE POWERFUL BUFFERS

Our belief systems provide us with the framework for our worldview, and they can offer powerful protection by buffering life's challenges. Already in our lives, we've experienced wounds that can alter how we see the world. I gave an example in chapter 7 about my toxic relationship with a coworker that forever changed my initial interactions with coworkers, making me more cautious and deliberate. My worldview shifted from the belief that coworkers are on the same team to the knowledge that not everyone wants others to succeed. My belief system helped me navigate this incident: I was able to forgive myself for trusting someone who didn't deserve my trust, and it allowed me to create new "rules" for evaluating relationships for warning signs or "red flags" and for honoring my ability to perceive those red flags.

It sounds so easy when I write the paragraph above, but the reality is that it took me several years to realize how much this relationship impacted me and my worldview. It took me a long time to realize that my core beliefs about trust had shifted based on this one relationship. That said, our belief systems reinforce how we see the world and help us to maintain biases that can impact our daily lives. Now when I meet new colleagues and coworkers, I tend to be cautious, but I don't default to the belief that people are out to sabotage me in some way. My worldview and belief system ensure that I am cautious in creating and maintaining relationships with others, and I generally believe that most people I meet are neutral or positive toward me (as I am toward them). If I had more cumulative negative experiences with coworkers (or others), I might have a negativity bias, in which I believed that others were "out to get me" and that no one could be trusted. I may well have earned this view based on my experiences, and it would likely change my outlook for the worse. There are many of us for whom this is a reality and being skeptical about others is a way of life, serving as protection from the realities that many midlife women have experienced.

Healing wounds that impact our core beliefs and worldview can take time and require help, such as through counseling, religious or spiritual guidance, disconnection from others, or some other path that is meaningful to the individual. Examining our wounds and processing how they have changed us for better and worse can be a powerful exercise in meeting ourselves where we are at this stage of our lives. We have never had the potential for as much wisdom or maturity as we do at this stage of our lives (the benefits of getting older!), and how we use this powerful knowledge to impact the next part of our lives is as important as the road that we took to get to the place we are today.

Some wounds may never fully heal, but this doesn't mean that they disconnect us from our belief systems or spiritual outlook. Indeed, these half-healed wounds are constant reminders of how we have changed in life and how our belief system helps guide us through our days. We can continue to strengthen our grounding in our belief systems through practices that help us connect to ourselves, others, and the world around us. These rituals can include religious and spiritual services, meditation, volunteer activities that serve other people or creatures, the practice of gratitude, physical activities, or being in nature. As we close this chapter, consider the reflection questions below to help you find deeper grounding in your belief systems and how these beliefs help you to navigate midlife.

REFLECTION

- Was there a time that your spiritual life helped you navigate a wound that you are still dealing with?
- What worked for you in that situation?
- How do you engage with those beliefs/behaviors in ways that are beneficial?
- How do you disengage with beliefs that no longer benefit you?
- How do you reconnect to yourself, others, and the world around you?
- What are some old practices that no longer serve you in midlife?
- What are some new practices that might help you going forward?

CONCLUSION

As I close this book and say goodbye, I'm struck by all the things that we didn't cover—there are so many things we could have explored! My hope—in the limited page space that we had together—is that you were able to discover tools and insights that help you. Ideally, completing the chapter exercises helped you to rediscover pieces of yourself, made you feel surer and more grounded, and allowed you to celebrate the refinement of yourself.

As you explored each chapter and considered the different facets of wellness and personal functioning, I hope that you have a better understanding of who you are and what you want for yourself at this phase of your life. Perhaps you were able to acknowledge some tension that has been building within you and found ways to release it because it no longer serves you. Maybe you let go of old habits because you found that they no longer served a function for the woman you are today. Ultimately, I hope that you are a woman who is closer to living your life on your terms versus the terms that don't work for you anymore.

Remember how we started this journey? It was with a story about my graduate school mentor commenting about how cautious I had become in recent years. I had become more comfortable, risk-averse, and had generally seemed to lose touch with the fearless young woman that I had been. That conversation swirled in my mind all day, leaving me feeling disoriented and unsure about the woman I had become. What were all these layers that had covered up the woman at my core? And how could I rediscover her? How would I even find her amid life, duties, and obligations? It felt as if I was struck with a sudden fever of questions that I couldn't get relief from. And yet the antidote was in my basement, waiting for me to find it.

You see, that conversation called to mind an image of me as a young girl. It was a very specific picture that I wanted, that I needed to find so I could see it firsthand. There in my basement was a scrapbook created by my mother with the image that I needed to see. It was a picture of me when I was about eight or nine years old, taken on a trip to New Jersey. In it, I am a messy, wild girl. The picture captures me on a swing set, kicking and yelling at the top of my lungs at the camera. The things I remember about this day: I am comfortable (literally: I'm wearing jeans, a T-shirt, and sneakers, the uniform of youth), I am unpretentious, I know my thoughts and will say anything to anyone, I am unselfconscious, I am powerful.

When I discussed the idea of "refinement" in chapter 1, I talked about it in terms of extracting a mineral from its natural source. This girl—this wild and free spirit who lets nothing stop her—is the purest mineral; she is the one with whom we lose touch as we get older. As I grow into my midlife, as I work to understand the power of this stage of my life, she is my guide. The questions that I ask myself are, *what would she do* and *how can I get closer to that brave and unbridled spirit?* I hope that every person reading this book has a mental picture that represents who they were before they started trying to live up to other people's expectations. I think that this quote from Jane Fonda captures the essence of this hope well.

> As I have gotten older, I have come back to where I started as that feisty girl who would climb to the top of the oak tree and lead armies up the hill and knew who she was and would stand up to anything and never told a lie. That part of a lot of girls goes way subterranean. It's not that it disappears. It doesn't get lost. It goes underground. And the goal of our lives is to bring her back up. (Demetrakas, 2018, 1:20:53)

Some of the most important attributes of that feisty girl who lives within us are that she knew her truth, she understood her values, and she understood her *value*. Our power in midlife is that we can embody all the dreams that our young selves imagined. Things that we didn't even dare to consider are available to us now. The transformation of our midlife and beyond isn't only about living well in this and future phases of our lives; it is about recapturing and honoring the perceptivity of our younger selves and living our values in ways that reflect the wisdom that we have collected through time. We do this by shaking off beliefs that others placed on us or that we created that are no longer valid, by living with boundaries that work for us, by caring for our physical bodies, nurturing our emotional selves, maintaining our most precious relationships, and creating legacies by doing the activities that mean the most to us and set us free.

I believe the path to "bring[ing] her back up" as Ms. Fonda stated, is wellness. It is getting back to basics, reflecting on the aspects of wellness that aid us in living our optimal lives and moving forward within those values that are true to who we are at this phase and stage of our lives. I encourage you to seek out a similar picture for inspiration, and if none exists, then create one for yourself. Look at this image often and use it as the inspiration to live powerfully, purposefully, and well. We all have a choice, choose wisely. I hope that you find a marriage between your unbridled self and the wise, refined woman within to live the most powerful life that you can.

REFERENCES

Arnett, J. (2018). Happily stressed: The complexity of well-being in midlife. *Journal of Adult Development, 25*(4), 270–278. https://doi.org/10.1007/s10804-018-9291-3

Barber, H. F. (1992). Developing strategic leadership: The US Army War College Experience. *The Journal of Management Development, 11*(6). https://doi.org/10.1108/02621719210018208

Barrett, D. (2016). Supernormal Stimuli. In Weekes-Shackelford, V., Shackelford, T., Weekes-Shackelford, V. (Eds.), *Encyclopedia of Evolutionary Psychological Science*. Springer. https://doi.org/10.1007/978-3-319-16999-6_94-1

Bateman, J. (2022). *Face: One square foot of skin*. Akashic Books.

Blume, J. (2001). *Are you there God? It's me, Margaret*. Atheneum Books for Young Readers.

Branscomb, A. W. (1995). Anonymity, autonomy, and accountability: Challenges to the First Amendment in cyberspaces. *The Yale Law Journal, 104*(7), 1639–1679. https://doi.org/10.2307/797027

Broderick, P. C., & Blewitt, P. (2006). Middle adulthood: Cognitive, personality, and social development. In *The life span: Human development for helping professionals* (2nd ed., pp. 404–441).

Brown, B. (2021). *Atlas of the heart*. Vermilion.

Brown, S. (2009). *Play: How it shapes the brain, opens the imagination, and invigorates the soul*. (C. C. Vaughan, Ed.). Penguin.

Burnett, B., & Evans, D. (2021). *Designing your new work life: How to thrive and change and find happiness and a new freedom at work*. Vintage.

Caldwell-Harris, Catherine. (2012). Understanding Atheism/non-belief as an expected individual-differences variable. *Religion, Brain & Behavior*. 2. 10.1080/2153599X.2012.668395.

Calhoun, A. (2020). *Why We Can't Sleep*. Grove Press.

Caputo, J., Pavalko, E. K., & Hardy, M. A. (2020). Midlife work and women's long-term health and mortality. *Demography, 57*(1), 373–402. https://doi.org/10.1007/s13524-019-00839-6

Childs, M. J. & Jones, A. (2023). Perceptions of individuals who engage in age concealment. *Evolutionary Behavioral Sciences, 17*(4), 407–419.

Christensen, J. (2023, November 15). WHO: Loneliness is a "growing public health concern" linked to social connection. CNN. https://www.cnn.com/2023/11/15/health/wholoneliness-social-connection/index.html

Clack, E. (2023). Everything Pamela Anderson has said about going makeup free after years of bombshell beauty. *People Magazine*. https://people.com/everything-pamela-anderson-has-said-about-her-makeup-free-moment-8362742

Demetrakas, J. (2018). *Feminists: What were they thinking?* Netflix.

Eklund, L., von Essen, E., Jonsson, F., & Johansson, M. (2022). Beyond a dichotomous understanding of online anonymity: Bridging the macro and micro level. *Sociological Research Online, 27*(2), 486–503. https://doi.org/10.1177/13607804211019760

Ephron, N. (2008). *I feel bad about my neck and other thoughts on being a woman*. Penguin Random House.

Falk, N. J. (2018). How to harness the untapped spending power of the 50-ish super consumer. *Forbes*. https://www.forbes.com/sites/njgoldston/2018/08/21/how-to-harness-the-untapped-spending-power-of-the-50-ish-super-consumer/?sh=5de0135416db

Farkas, C., Ziegler, G., Meretei, A., & Lörincz, A. (2002). Anonymity and accountability in self-organizing electronic communities. *WPES '02: Proceedings of the 2002 ACM workshop on Privacy in the Electronic Society*. https://doi.org/10.1145/644527.644536

Feeney, J., & Noller, P. (1996). Adult attachment (Vol. 14). Sage.

Feskens, E. J. M., Bailey, R., Bhutta, Z., Biesalski, H.-K., Eicher-Miller, H., Kramer, K., Pan, W.-H., Griffiths, J. C. (2022). Women's health: Optimal nutrition throughout the lifecycle. *European Journal of Nutrition, 61*, 1–23. https://link.springer.com/article/10.1007/s00394-022-02915-x

Gallup. (2023). *Religion*. https://news.gallup.com/poll/1690/Religion.aspx

Giordano, A. (2021). *The clinical guide to treating behavioral addictions*. Springer.

Gittleman, M. (2022). The "Great Resignation" in perspective. *Monthly Labor Review*. U.S. Bureau of Labor Statistics. https://doi.org/10.21916/mlr.2022.20

Goldenberg, I., Stanton, M., & Goldenberg, H. (2017). *Family therapy: An overview* (9th ed.). Cengage Learning.

Haan, K. (2023). Remote work statistics and trends in 2024. *Forbes*. https://www.forbes.com/advisor/business/remote-work-statistics/#sources_section

Hall, R. L. (2007). On the move: Exercise, leisure activities, and midlife women. In J. C. Chrisler & D. McCreary (Eds.), *Handbook of gender research in psychology: Gender research in general and experimental psychology* (pp. 79–94). Springer.

Harahap, R. K., & Daulay, A. A. (2023). Toxic parenting and its impact on children's language ethics. *Counsenesia Indonesian Journal of Guidance and Counseling, 4*(1), 41–52.

Hare, N. (2022, September 1). What is "quiet quitting" and how should leaders respond? *Forbes.* https://www.forbes.com/sites/allbusiness/2022/09/01/what-is-quiet-quitting-and-how-should-leaders-respond/?sh=7cc6f0bc6de0

Haynes, T., & Clements, R. (2018). Dopamine, smartphones & you: A battle for your time. *Harvard Science in the News.* https://sitn.hms.harvard.edu/flash/2018/dopaminesmartphones-battle-time/

Hayward, R. D., Krause, N., Ironson, G., & Pargament, K. I. (2016). Externalizing religious health beliefs and health and well-being outcomes. *Journal of Behavioral Medicine, 39*, 887–895. https://doi.org/10.1007/s10865-016-9761-7

Higgins, C. (2005). Dewey's conception of vocation: Existential, aesthetic, and educational implications for teachers. *Journal of Curriculum Studies, 37*(4), 441–464. https://doi.org/10.1080/00220270500048502

Hoffower, H., & Kiersz, A. (2021, September 22). Millennials make more money than any other generation did at their age but are way less wealthy. The affordability crisis is to blame. *Insider.* https://www.businessinsider.com/millennials-highest-earning-generation-less-wealthy-boomers-2021-9

Holahan, C., Holahan, C., Velasquez, K., Jung, S., North, R., & Pahl, S. (2011). Purposiveness and leisure-time physical activity in women in early midlife. *Women & Health, 51*(7), 661–675. https://doi.org/10.1080/03630242.2011.617811

Infurna, F. J., Gerstorf, D., & Lachman, M. E. (2020). Midlife in the 2020s: Opportunities and challenges. *The American Psychologist, 75*(4), 470–485. https://doi.org/10.1037/amp0000591

Infurna, F. J., Staben, O. E., Gardner, M. J., Grimm, K. J., & Luthar, S. S. (2023). The accumulation of adversity in midlife: Effects on depressive symptoms, life satisfaction, and character strengths. *Psychology and Aging, 38*(3), 230–246. https://doi.org/10.1037/pag0000725

Jaffe, S. (2023, May 13). US surgeon general: Loneliness is a public health crisis. *The Lancet, 401.* https://www.thelancet.com/article/S0140-6736(23)01234-X/fulltext

James, K., Verplanken, B., & Rimes, K. A. (2015). Self-criticism as a mediator in the relationship between unhealthy perfectionism and distress. *Personality and Individual Differences, 79*, 123–128.

Kabat-Zinn, J. (2013). *Full catastrophe living.* Bantam.

Kagan, R., Shiozawa, A., Epstein, A., & Espinosa, R. (2021). Impact of sleep disturbances on employment and work productivity among midlife women in the US SWAN database: A brief report. *Menopause, 28*(10), 1176–1180. https://doi.org/10.1097/GME.0000000000001834

Koenig, H. G., King, D. E., & Carson, V. B. (2012). *Handbook of religion and health* (2nd ed.). New York: Oxford University Press.

Lewis, T., Amini, F., & Lannon, R. (2001). *A general theory of love*. Vintage Books.

Marks, E. (2021). Regina King. *British Vogue*. https://www.vogue.co.uk/arts-and-lifestyle/article/regina-king-interview

Matthews, K. A., Kravitz, H. M., Lee, L., Harlow, S. D, Bromberger, J. T., Joffe, H., & Hall, M. H. (2020). Does midlife aging impact women's sleep duration, continuity, and timing? A longitudinal analysis from the Study of Women's Health Across the Nation. *Sleep, 43*(4). https://doi.org/10.1093/sleep/zsz259

McEwen, B. S. & Stellar, E. (1993). Stress and individual: Mechanisms leading to disease. *Arch Intern Medicine, 153*(18), 2093–2101, https://doi.org/10.1001/archinte.1993.00410180039004

Meshi, D., & Ellithorpe, M. E. (2021). Problematic social media use and social support received in real-life versus on social media: Associations with depression, anxiety and social isolation. *Addictive Behaviors, 119*, 106949–106949.

Miller, L. (2017). The ambition collision. *The Cut*. https://www.thecut.com/2017/09/what-happens-to-ambition-in-your-30s.html

Moyer, A. E., Rodin, J. Grilo, C. M., Cummings, N., Larson, L. M., & Rebuffe-Scrive, M. (1994). Stress-induced cortisol response and fat distribution in women. *Obesity Research, 2*(3), 255–262. https://doi.org/10.1002/j.1550-8528.1994.tb00055.x

Myers, J. E., & Sweeney, T. J. (2004). The indivisible self: An evidenced-based model of wellness. *The Journal of Individual Psychology, 60*(3), 234–244.

Oliveira, E., Kim, H. S., Lacroix, E., de Fatima Vasques, M., Durante, C. R., Pereira, D., Cabral, J. R., Bernstein, P. S., Garcia, X., Ritchie, E. V., & Tavares, H. (2020). The clinical utility of food addiction: Characteristics and psychosocial impairments in a treatment-seeking sample. *Nutrients, 12*(11), 3388–. https://doi.org/10.3390/nu12113388

Østby, K. A., Mykletun, A., & Nilsen, W. (2018). Explaining the gender gap in sickness absence. *Occupational Medicine, 68*(5), 320–326. https://doi.org/10.1093/occmed/kqy062

Pargament K. I. (2011). Religion and coping: The current state of knowledge. In Folkman S. (ed.), *Oxford Handbook of Stress, Health, and Coping*, New York, Oxford University Press.

Parker, K., & Wang, W. (2013, March 14). Modern parenthood: Roles of moms and dads converge as they balance work and family. *Pew Research Center*. https://www.pewresearch.org/social-trends/2013/03/14/modern-parenthood-roles-ofmoms-and-dads-converge-as-they-balance-work-and-family/#chapter-6-time-in-work-and-leisure-patterns-by-gender-and-family-structure.

Prochaska, J. O., & Norcross, J. C. (2001). Stages of change. *Psychotherapy, 38*(4), 443–448. https://doi.org/10.1037/0033-3204.38.4.443

Rubinstein, H. R., & Foster, J. L. H. (2013). "I don't know whether it is to do with age or to do with hormones and whether it is to do with a stage in your life": Making sense of menopause and the body. *Journal of Healthy Psychology, 18*(2), 292–307. https://doi.org/10.1177/1359105312454040

Samson, N., Fink, B., Matts, P. J., Dawes, N. C., & Weitz, S. (2010). Visible changes of female facial skin surface topography in relation to age and attractiveness perception. *Journal of Cosmetic Dermatology, 9*(2), 79–88. https://doi.org/10.1111/j.1473-2165.2010.00489.x

Savci, M. & Aysan, F. (2017). Technological addictions and social connectedness: Predictor effect of internet addiction, social media addiction, digital game addiction and smartphone addiction on social connectedness. *The Journal of Psychiatry and Neurological Sciences*, 30, 202–216.

Schaal, M. L., Lee, W., Egger, M. J., Nygaard, I. E, & Shaw, J. M. (2016). Physical activity patterns in healthy middle-aged women. *Journal of Women Aging, 28*(6), 469–476.

Scharfe, E., Pitman, R., & Cole, V. (2017). Function of attachment hierarchies in young adults experiencing the transition from university. *Interpersonal: An International Journal on Personal Relationships, 11*(1), 40–54. https://doi.org/10.5964/ijpr.v11i1.223

Sharf, R. S. (2012). *Theories of psychotherapy and counseling: Concepts and cases* (5th ed.). Brooks/Cole Cengage Learning.

Sirgy, M. J., Uysal, M., & Kruger, S. (2017). Towards a benefits theory of leisure well-being. *Applied Research in Quality of Life, 12*(1), 205–228. https://doi.org/10.1007/s11482-016-9482-7

Soares, J. J. F., Grossi, G., & Sundin, Ö. (2007). Burnout among women: Associations with demographic/socio-economic, work, lifestyle, and health factors. *Archives of Women's Mental Health, 10*, 61–71.

Stalp, M. C., Radina, M. E., & Lynch, A. (2008). "We do it cuz it's fun": Gendered fun and leisure for midlife women through Red Hat Society Membership. *Sociological Perspectives, 51*(2), 325–348. https://doi.org/10.1525/sop.2008.51.2.325

Stevenson, R. J. (2017). Psychological correlates of habitual diet in healthy adults. *Psychological Bulletin, 143*(1), 53–90.

Stoeber, J. & Otto, K. (2006). Positive conceptions of perfectionism: Approaches, evidence, challenges. *Personality and Social Psychology Review, 10*(4), 295–319.

Thomas, A. J., Mitchell, E. S., & Woods, N. F. (2018). The challenges of midlife women: Themes from the Seattle midlife women's health study. *Women's Midlife Health, 4*(8). https://doi.org/10.1186/s40695-018-0039-9

Tsipursky, G. (2023, February 18). How associations can improve new member retention. *Forbes.* https://www.forbes.com/sites/glebtsipursky/2023/02/18/how-associations-can-improve-new-member-retention/?sh=1c92dc653216

US Bureau of Labor Statistics (2023). *Women in the labor force: A databook.* https://www.bls.gov/opub/reports/womens-databook/2022/home.htm

US Census Bureau. (2020). *United States marriage and divorce rates declined in the last 10 years.* Census.gov. https://www.census.gov/library/stories/2020/12/unitedstates-marriage-and-divorce-rates-declined-last-10-years.html

Wolfe, W. L., & Yakabovits, L. (2024). I'll see your beautified photo and raise you one: An experimental investigation of the effect of edited social media photo exposure. *Psychology of Popular Media, 13*(2), 249–255. https://doi.org/10.1037/ppm0000443

World Health Organization. (2019, May 28). Burn-out an "occupational phenomenon": International Classification of Diseases. https://www.who.int/news/item/28-05-2019-burn-out-an-occupational-phenomenon-international-classification-of-diseases#:~:text=It%20is%20characterized%20by%20three%20dimensions%3Afeeling%20of%20energy,evidence-based%20guidelines%20on%20mental%20wellbeing%20in%20the%20workplace

Yamada, H. (2023). Madonna responds to "ageism" after comments on her appearance at the Grammys. *ABC News.* https://abcnews.go.com/GMA/Culture/madonna-responds-ageism-after-comments-appearance-grammys/story?id=96963896

Zivnuska, S., Carlson, J. R., Carlson, D. S., Harris, R. B., & Harris, K. J. (2019). Social media addiction and social media reactions: The implications for job performance. *The Journal of Social Psychology, 159*(6), 746–760. https://doi.org/10.1080/00224545.2019.1578725

INDEX

abuse, 16–17, 107–8, 132–33, 184
acceptance, xiv, 86, 88, 139
accessibility, 127, 135–39
accountability, 49, 190; social relationships and, 127, 130–34, 139; toxic relationships and, 109–12
acne, 77–78
activity, physical, 71–73
addiction, social media, 11, 126
adolescence, teenage years and, 77, 133, 164, 182, 191; decreased social connectedness among, 126; puberty in, 59, 90; values and, 27
adulthood, 83, 89, 95–96, 167, 187; early, ix, xiv, 90, 182
advancement opportunities, workplace, 149
adverse experiences, management of, 189–90
aesthetics, 177
affairs, emotional, 103
agape (selfless love), 98
age concealment, 77–78
age spots, 84, 89
aging populations, 147
agnosticism, 182–83, 188
AI-enhanced images, 82
alcohol, 8, 67, 69–70
allostatic load, 58–61
ambiguity, 43–45, 48, 62–65

ambivalence, 48
Amini, F., 126
Amy (dietician), 69–70
Anderson, Pamela, 89
androgen, 80
angst, existential, viii, 6–7, 47–48
Aniston, Jennifer, 32–33
anonymity, 127, 131, 133–35, 139
anorexia nervosa, 71
antiaging treatments, 78
anticipation, 98
antidepressants, 39–40
anti-inflammatory foods, 68–69
antisocial behavior, 134
anxiety, 11, 13, 46, 48, 123–24, 136, 150; children experiencing, 107; health and, 56; perfectionism and, 63
appearances, aging and, 23–25, 77, 92–93; internal validation and, 78–79; science and, 80–83; stages of realization regarding, 83–91
Are You There God? It's Me, Margaret (Blume), 87
arthritis, 59, 84
Artist/Creator play personality, 169–70
ASERVIC. *See* Association for Spiritual, Ethical, and Religious Values in Counseling
ashram, 1, 78–79

INDEX

Association for Spiritual, Ethical, and Religious Values in Counseling (ASERVIC), 182
assumptions, 152
atheism, 182–83, 188
attachment theory, 106–7
attention, 109, 137–38
attractiveness, 78, 82
autonomy, vii, xvii, 35–36, 107, 127, 142–43, 155–57
autopilot, 124
awkwardness, viii
Aysan, F., 126

baby face, 83
baptism, Catholic, 181
barriers: language, 129; to leisure, 174–76, 178; to social engagement, 165, 190
Bateman, Justine, 87–88
bedtime, 37, 66–67
behavioral goals, 74
belief systems, beliefs and, 2, 15, 27, 31–32, 45, 108, 181–83; buffering provided by, 196–97; development of, 185–88; flexibility of, 33; health and, 188–91; "I Am" exercise and, 184, *184–85*; in intimate relationships, *101*, 101–2, *102*; irrational, 13–14; meaning and, 191–93; physical health and, 57; social relationships and, *121–22*; values and, 41–42
belonging, sense of, 107, 126
benchmarks, 23, 154
betrayal, double, 194
biases, 150, 196
"big T" trauma, 193–94

binge eating, 8–9, 18, 71
biological changes, xi, 80, 124
biological relationships, 98, 109
birds, 81–82
birthrates, 147
blame, 2, 18, 109, 150
blood, 60, 87
blood pressure, 60–61m 68
Blume, Judy, 87
body doubles, 82
body positivity, 90
The Book of Boundaries (Urban), 155–56
Boomer generation, 3–5
boredom, 118, 159
boundaries, 2, 14, 17, 37–38, 42, 67, 99, 138; in intimate relationships, *101*, 101–3, *102*, 112–13, 116; physical health and, 57, 74–75; social relationship, *121–22*; workplace, 33–36, 148, 154–56, 158
Bowlby, John, 106
brains, 10, 22, 46–47, 66–67, 126
bravery, courage and, 48–50, 104–5, 158
breast cancer, 55–56
breathing, breath and, 21–22
Brown, Brené, 62
Brown, S., 167–69, 176
buccal fat removal, 83
bulimia nervosa, 71
bullying, 132, 193
Bureau of Labor Statistics, United States, 7
Burnett, Bill, 152–53, 158
burnout, 142–44, 146–52, *160*
busyness, 14, 75, 117, 141, 149
bystander intervention, 131–32

caffeine, 67, 74–75
Calhoun, Ada, 4
call outs, 131–32
calories, 69–70
Canada, 163
"cancel culture," 132–33
cancer, 55–56, 86–87
candy stripers, hospital, 191–92
careers, 4–5, 7, 24–25, 141–43, 145, *145–46*, 149, 152. *See also* vocations; workplace
caregiving, caregivers and, 39, 45, 147, 149
Casey (nonprofit worker), xii–xiii, 27
Cass (coworker), 158
Catholicism, 129, 181–82
cautiousness, vii, 199
celebrities, 32–33, 82, 89, 132
cellulite, 84
changes, xi–xii, 18–19, 58–59, 104, 124, 157; appearances and, 86, 92–93
chemical imbalances, 13
chemical payoffs, 137–38
childhood, youth and, 4, 59, 83, 87, 143, 167, 200–201; leisure time and, 163–64, 169–70, *171–72*; moral development in, 186; religion and, 181–82
children, 15–16, 98, 147, 174–75, 190–92; attachment theory and, 106–7
China, 129–30
cholesterol, 61
Christianity, 98
chronic stress, 146–47
circadian rhythms, 67
civil rights movement, 3, 187

clothing, shopping for, 88
code-switching, 27
coffee, 74–75
cognitive immersion, 164
cohabiting partnerships, nonmarried, 97
"cola wars" (1980s), 132–33
collagen, 80–81, 87
Collector play personality, 169
comfort, ix, 109, 186, 199–200
commitments, 128
common good, 187
communication, 36–37, 110, 117, 135–36, 155; boundary, 43; honest and, *101*, 103–4; nonverbal, 79, 134; sarcasm and, 7
communities, 50, 116, 132; belief, 15, 174, 182, 189–90, 194–95; online, 133–34; self-control in, 190
compartmentalization, 143
compassion, 64, 133
Competitor play personality, 168
complacency, 17
complexity, 43–45, 48
condescension, 85
confirmation, Catholic, 181
conflicts, 95, 117, 119, 127, 139
Confucianism, 129
confusion, 181–82
connectedness, sense of, 126, 137, 185
conscience, 186
consciousness, 186
consent, 138
control, xvii, 40, 49, 58, 87, 108, 120; parental, 107; physical health and, 62–63
conversion, religious, 129

coping, 5–8, 48, 61; belief systems and, 189–90; with death, 39; healthy, 8, 18; leisure activities and, 171
Corn, Seane, 85–86
cortisol secretion, 60
costs: of living, 4–5; medical care, 58
counseling, xv–xvii, 42, 112, 152, 182–83, 186, 191; for burnout, 147; family, 16, 36–37; for internal and external stressors, 47–48; marriage, 110
"courtly love," 97
COVID-19 pandemic, 8, 34, 43–45, 66, 72, 113, 125, 148, 150
coworkers, 100, *121*, 131, 196, 228
crises, midlife, 1, 5, 109
criticism, 63–64, 107
cross-cultural exchanges, 129–30
cruelty, 134
crying, 39–40, 105, 113
curiosity, 89, 134
cynical humor, 6–7, 146

death, xv, 8, 39–40, 110, 113
"deathbed regrets," 164
decision making, 22, 98, 104, 142; Eisenhower decision matrix, 40, *50*, 50–53, *51*, *52*; informed, 61
deindividuation, 134
delegation, *51*
demands, work, 147–49
denial, 11–12, 56, 84–87
depression, 10–11, 13, 47, 118, 124, 150, 170
dermatology, 77–78
Designing Your Work Life (Burnett, Evans), 152–53
desirability, 11–12, 79

desires, 48, 72, 98, 123, 132
development, midlife, xi
Dewey, John, 144
dietetics, 69–70
diffuse boundaries, 37
Director play personality, 168–69
disability benefits, 158
disagreement: harmonious, 128–31, 139, 183; religious, 183
discomfort, viii–ix, xii, 2–3
discrimination, 149
disembodiment, 134
disempowerment, 88
disengagement, relationship, 108
disillusionment, 149
dismissiveness, 85, 107
dissatisfaction, job, 159–60
distractions, 9–10, 14, 166
distress, emotional, 63–65, 107
disturbances, sleep, 65–67
divorce, 97, 123, 133, 181, 194
dopamine, 137–38
double betrayal, 194–95
drug use, 8

early adulthood, ix, xiv, 90, 182
eating disorders, 8–9, 14, 18, 71
economic benefits, leisure and, 176–77
education, x, 5, 28, 35, 83, 154, 170, 181–82, 191
eggs, birds and, 81–82
egocentrism, egos and, 35, 111
Eisenhower decision matrix, 40, *50*, 50–53, *51*, *52*
Ellis, Albert, 13
email, 133; work, 39, 154–56
emotional abuse, 108, 132–33
emotional affairs, 103

emotional distress, 63–65, 107
emotional labor, 7, 148–49, 191
emotional needs, 103
emotional relationships, 71, 103
emotional support, 45, 125, 131, 207
empathy, 107, 126, 134
employment *vs.* occupation, 142–43, *145–46*, 145–47. *See also* workplace
empowerment, 86–87, 90–91, 112
endocrine system, 59–60
endorphins, 9
energy, 69–70, 120
environmental issues, 47–48
Ephron, Nora, 92–93
equity, 186–87
eros (romantic love), 97–98
escape, sense of, 176–77
estrogen, 68, 80–81
ethics, 130; of anonymity, 134; of care, 191; universal, 186–87
eudaemonic well-being, 165–67
evaluating relationships, 196
Evans, Dave, 152–53, 158
evolution, individual, xi–xii, 104–5, 130
exercise, physical, 32–33, 59, 63–64, 84
exercises: aging and appearance, 91–92; decision matrix, *52*, 52–53; global assessment of wellness, 23–25; "I Am" poem, 184, *184–85*; inner circle, *102*; intimate relationship, 113, *114–15*; leisure related, *172*, 172–73, 178–79; physical wellness, 57–58; social relationship, 119, *119*, *121–22*; values reflection, 41–42; values sort, 29–30; vocational

satisfaction, 159–60, *159–60*; work-life balance, 144–45, *145–46*, *161*
exhaustion, xiii, 1, 12, 95, 146, 149
existential angst, viii, 6–7, 47–48
existentialism, 182–83, *184*
expectations, vii, xv, 63; around appearances, 82, 87–89; of children, 107; gendered, 28; of others, 200–201; workplace, 155
Explorer play personality, 168
expression, freedom of, 131
external stressors, 40, 47–49, 60–61, 123–24
external validation, 79
extroversion, extroverts and, 177

Face (Bateman), 87–88
Facebook, 133, 141
face-to-face interaction, 125
facial age concealment, 77–78
failure, feelings of, vii, ix, 63, 107, 123, 150–51
family therapy, counseling and, 16, 36–37
fantasies: about growing up, 83; about quitting, 157–58
fatigue, 66, 149–50, 160, 174
fearlessness, vii, 199
fear of missing out (FOMO), 138, 155
fears, viii, 17, 63, 106–7, 141
feet, arthritic, 59, 84
Feminine Mystique (Friedan), 3
femininity, xi
feminism, second wave, 3
"fight or flight" responses, 22, 46–47, 60
filters, images and, 82

financial independence, 3
financial planners, 157
firstborn children, 16
flash mob–style dance, 71–73
flexibility, *121*, 152–53, 156, 158–59, 173; of beliefs, 33; of boundaries, 37
flirting, 79
flow state, 164
FOMO. *See* fear of missing out
Fonda, Jane, 200–201
food, 37–38, 67; eating disorders and, 8–9, 14, 18, 71; emotional relationships with, 71; inflammation and, 63, 68–70
forgiveness, 133, 194–96
Fowler, James, 187
Fowler's stages of faith development, 186–88
fragility, emotional, 108
France, 97
freedom, viii, 89, 131
free speech, 131
free time, 109
Friedan, Betty, 3
friends, friendship and, 87, 107, 112–13, 117–18, *121*
frog in boiling water analogy, 106, 114
frown lines, 84
frustration, 34, 64, 143
fulfillment, sense of, 1, 5, 7, 123, 170–71; social relationships and, 126–27; vocations and, 142, 144

GAF Scale, 22. *See* Global Assessment of Functioning
gallows humor, 6–7, 146

GAW. *See* Global Assessment of Wellness
gender, 11, 18, 62, 79–80, 85, 88–89; barriers to leisure and, 174–76, 178; belief systems and, 189; burnout and, 147–51; education and, 5; emotional labor and, 191; expectations and, 28; hormonal changes and, 80
generational bridging, 4–5, 147
genetics, 46, 60–61
Gen X, 4–5, 147
Germany, 163
"ghost tigers," 47, 60
Giordano, Amanda, 126
"glass ceilings," 3–4
Global Assessment of Functioning (GAF) Scale, 22
Global Assessment of Wellness (GAW), 41
global public health concern, loneliness as a, 10, 117–18
God, higher powers and, 181–83, *184*, 190, 194
"going postal" (phrase), 7
Google, 138
gossip, 132, 150
gratitude, 112
gray hairs, 83
Great Resignation, 157
grief, 39–40, 51, *51*, 96
group mentalities, 134–35
guilt, 165

habits, 9, 31–32, 69, 199
hair, 81, 83
happiness, 59, 143
hardships, 105, 191–92
harm, 184

harmonious disagreement, 128–31, 139, 183
hate groups, online, 135
Hayward, R. D., 189
healing, trauma and, 194–97
health, *101*, 113, 123–24; belief systems and, 188–91; eating disorders impacting, 8–9, 14, 18, 71; emotional, 40–45; leisure and, 166, 174, 176, 178; mental, xvii–xviii, 11–13, 23–25, 40–45, 90, 109, 137, 156–58, 160; personal, 5, 34, 190; psychological, 166, 189; social, 24, 117–19, 127, 139; work and, 144, 147, 150
health, physical, 23–25, 32–33, 57–64, 158, 166; early detection, 55–56; food and, 68–71; movement and, 71–73; sleep and, 65–67
health insurance, 56, 58
healthy coping, 8, 18
healthy relationships, *121*
heartbreak, 96
heart disease, 61, 68
help, asking for, 49–50, *51*, 51–53, 110
Higgins, C., 144
higher education, 28, 35, 83, 154
high-impact workouts, 32–33, 59
homeostasis, 15
honesty, *101*, 103–4, *121*
hope, 96
hormonal changes, xi, 58, 68, 80, 174
hospitals, 58, 113, 191–92
"how healthy is your pond?" exercise, 113, *114–15*
human development, ix
human rights, 182
humiliation, 107, 132

humor, cynical, 6–7, 146
hurtful behaviors, 134
hygiene, sleep, 66
hyperpalatable foods, 82
"hysteria," 11

"I Am" exercise, 184, *184–85*
ICD catalog. *See* International Classifications of Disease
identity, 65, 78, 92, 134
I Feel Bad about My Neck and Other Thoughts on Being a Woman (Ephron), 92–93
illness, xv, 56, 68, 158
image-editing tools, 82
imagery, self-imagery and, 71, 82, 194, 200
imagination, 169
immersion, cognitive, 164
immune system, 59–60
impulsivity, 2
income, viii, 4–5, 17, 104, 144, 149, 153, 158
incongruence, 12–13
independence, 3, 88, 107, 147
individualism, 147
individuality, 169
individual rights, 1, 186
"Indivisible Self" (wellness model), xv–xvi
indoctrination, 14–15
inevitability, 85, 93
infants, 106
infatuation, 98
inflammation, 60, 81; food and, 63, 68–70
inflation, 148
influence, sphere of, 127
informed decisions, 61

inner critics, 63–65, 75
insomnia, 66
Instagram, 11, 133
instincts, institutional knowledge and, 81–82, 147
insurance, health, 56
internalizations, 78, 123, 138, 187; around beliefs, 14, 46, 192–93; expectations and, 88–89; instinctual, 81–82; around shame, 62; of social messaging, 16–17; of trauma, 194
internal responsibilities, 51–53
internal stressors, 40, 45–49
internal validation, 79, 93
International Classifications of Disease (ICD) catalog, 146–47
internet, 126, 136. *See also* virtual worlds, online networks
intersectionality, 4
intimate relationships, intimacy and, 17, 23–25, 118; "how healthy is your pond?" exercise, 113, *114–15*; inner circle and, 99–102, *100*, *101*, *102*, 111–12, 119, *119*; keystones of, 103–6; love and, 96–99; reflection questions, 102, 116; toxicity in, 106–11
intrinsic value, 166
introspection, 159
introversion, introverts and, 177
irrational beliefs, 13–14
isolation, 8, 41, 107, 136

James, K., 64
jaw tension, 21
jealousy, 98, 106, 109
Jesuit priests, 129
Joker play personality, 168

Journal of Women Aging, 72
judgment, feelings of, 183
junk food, 82

kayaking, 175–76
kindergarten, 181–82
kindness, 42, *101*, *121*, 131
Kinesthetic play personality, 168, 170
Kohlberg, Lawrence, 186–87
Kohlberg's stages of moral development, 186–87

language: barriers, 129; code-switching, 27; play, *171–72*, 172–73
Lannon, R., 126
laugh lines, 83
leadership roles, workplace, 149, 152, 157
legislative rights, 4
leisure, free time and, 24, 165–66, 177–79; barriers to, 174–76, 178; childhood experiences of, 160–70, *171–72*; midlife, 169–71, *171–72*, 173; play and, 167–70, *171–73*, 172–73
Lewis, T., 126
limbic resonance, 126, 134, 137
lines, facial wrinkles and, 77–78, 83–84, 87
listening, viii, 79, *101*, *121*
"little t" trauma, 193–94
loneliness, 10, 41, 107, 117–18
long-distance phone calls, 136
long-term, 105, 124; exposure to stress, 60; relationships, 108, 112–13; risks, 68

INDEX 217

love, 95, *121*, 143, 190, 194;
   families and, 15–16; intimate
   relationships and, 96–99, 113;
   self, xiv; shame and, 62
loyalty, 128–29
ludus (playful love), 98

Madonna, 89–80
makeup, 10, 83–84, 86
malaise, 6
mammograms, 55–56
mania (obsessive love), 98
marginalized groups, 4, 131
marriage, viii, 1, 6, 100, 109–10;
   divorce and, 5, 97, 181, 194;
   trauma relating to, 194
"masking," social, 120
mass shootings, 7
McEwen, B. S., 59–60
meaningful connections, 118
meaning-making, meaning and,
   166; belief systems and, 191–93;
   existential, 167; vocational, 144
medical professionals, 13, 39–40, 53,
   55–56, 62–63, 73
meditation, 1
membership organizations, 123–25
memes, 10, 125, 136, 141
menopause, xi, 58–59, 68, 80, 174
Menopause (journal), 65
menstrual cycles, 58, 87
mental health, xvii–xviii, 11–13,
   23–25, 40–45, 90, 109, 137,
   156–58, 160
mentors, vii–viii, xi, 149, 199
metabolism, 58, 68
metrics, success, 152–54, 158
microaggressions, 149
micromanaging, 157

microneedling, 87
middle children, 16
middle-class women, white, 3–4
midlife, women. *See specific topics*
Millennials, 4, 147
mindset, 62
mineral extraction metaphor, xiii,
   200
minority status, 4
miscommunications, 127
mistrust, 157
"mob mentality," 134–35
"Moon River" (song), 95–96
morals, morality and, 177, 182;
   development of, 186–88
mosquito bite metaphor, 45
motivation, motives and, 13, 18,
   48, 72, 141, 144; self, 53, 167;
   ulterior, 127
mourning *vs.* embracing, stage of
   realization, 86–87
movement, physical, 71–73
muscles, 32–33, 58, 63, 68, 84;
   breathing and, 21–22
mutual trust, *121*
Myers, J. E., xv–xvi
"MyPlate" (food pyramid), USDA,
   69

narcissism, 78, 109, 111
needs, 7, 15; emotional, 103;
   personal, 159
negative coping mechanisms, 7–9
negative religious coping, 190
negative self-talk, 64, 82
negative thoughts, 150
negativity bias, 150
neglect, 107
nervous system, 22

neurology, 59–60
"New Coke" campaign, 132–33
nicotine, 67
1984 (Orwell), 135
nonbelief, nonreligious belief systems and, 182–83, 188–91
nonconformity, 41
nonprofits, xii–xiii
nonverbal, 79, 134
norms, social, ix, 7, 127, 131
North Carolina, 1
notifications, dopamine and, 138
nutrition, 37–38

obligations, duties and, 123, 138, 164–65, 173
occupation *vs.* employment, 142–43, 145–46, 145–47
Oklahoma, 7
online hate groups, 135
orthopedic health, 87
Orwell, George, 135
outer social circles, 119, *119*
overcorrections, social, 132

pain, 55, 62, 68–69
"painkiller" hormone (endorphins), 9
parasocial relationships, 118
parents, caregivers and, 1, 95–96, 98, *101*, 136–38, 190–92; aging and, viii, 88; attachment theory and, 106; death of, 39, 110, 113; divorce and, 181; leisure and, 163–64; narcissistic, 109; religion and, 181–82; social messaging by, 16; toxic, 106–7
Pargament, Ken, 190
Paris Fashion Week, 89

partners, partnership status and, 6, 17, *101*, 103, 108–9, 123
passion, 98
pediatrics units, hospital, 191–92
pedometers, 73
people-pleasing, 138
Pepsi, 132–33
perceptions, 122–23, 129; around appearances, 77–91; around wellness, 22–25
perfectionism, 4, 13–14, 58, 63–64
perimenopause, xi, 58, 68
periods (menses), 58, 87
permeability, in boundaries, 37
personal health, 5, 34, 190
personality development, 126
personality types, play, 168–70, *171–72*, 172–73
philautia (self-love), 99
philia (affectionate love), 98
phone calls, long-distance, 136
photo editing, 82
physical abuse, 107
physical desire, 98
physiology, 60, 68
Piaget, Jean, 186
plasma, blood, 87
platelet-rich plasma facials (PRPs), 87
play, 166–70, *171–72*, 172–73
poetry, 184, *184–85*
polarization, 45, 133
popular culture, xvi, 82
pornography, 82
portion sizes, food, 69–70
positivity, toxic, 150
pottery, 175
power, 11, 38, 90, 132–33, 135; of beliefs and habits, 32; of family, 14–17; in midlife, 200

pragma (enduring love), 98
pragmatism, 159
preoccupations, 71, 107
Pretty Woman (film), 82
preventative care, 56, 62
priorities, 27, 75, 153; belief systems and, 186; decision matrix and, *50, 51*, 51–52; values and, xiii, 29–31
privilege, 1
protein, 68–70
PRPs. *See* platelet-rich plasma facials
psychoanalysis, 11
psychological health, 166, 189
psychotherapy, 13, 193
puberty, 59, 90
public life, 118, 120
public shaming, online, 132
Purche, W. R., 130
purpose: existential, 165–66; sense of, 144, 151, 161, 166

"quiet quitting," 150, 157
quitting, 64, 123; fantasies about, 157–58; "quiet," 150, 157

rationalizations, 40
reading, 173
real-life interactions, 118, *121*, 125–27, 130–31, 134–37, 139–40
real-time video chats, 136
reciprocal relationships, 97, 101, 152
recreational therapy, 169–70
Reddit, 133–34
refinement, personal, xiii–xv, 199–200
reflection questions, 53; appearance related, 80, 91–92; belief system, 195, 197; intimate relationship, 102, 116; leisure related, 178; social relationship, 120, 139–40; values related, 31; vocation related, 160–61
reframes, 152
regrets, 92–93, 164
rejection, 107
relationships. *See* social relationships
release, tension, 199
religions, religious doctrines and, 14–15, 129, 181–83; coping tools and, 190; "I Am" exercise and, 184, *184–85*. *See also* belief systems
reproductive rights, 3
research librarians, 165
resentment, 6, 149
resilience, 13
resourcefulness, 13
respect, 27–28, 35–36, 130, 187
responsibilities, xv, 1, 49, 107, 130–31, 142, 174; adulthood and, 83, 89; caregiving, 147, 149; decision matrix and, *51*, 51–53; fulfillment and, 7; in toxic relationships, 109–12; work, 155. *See also* obligations, duties and
restlessness, sense of, 143
retention rates, membership, 124–25
retirement savings, 157
Ricci, Matteo, 129–30
rights, 4; civil, 3, 187; of free speech, 131; human, 182; individual, 1, 186; voting, 187
rigidity, 32–33, 37–38, 167
Rimes, K. A., 64
risk-taking, vii–viii, 61, 134, 167
Roberts, Julia, 82
rock bottom, 8–11
rock climbing, 63

romantic love and relationships, 97–98, 108–10
rural areas, 136

sabbaticals, workplace, 152
sabotage, xiii, 89, 196
sacrifice, 15, 98, 190
sadness, 110
safety, xii, 17, 175–76; vulnerability and, 105
sandwich generation, 147
sarcasm, 6–7, 146
satisfaction: mental health and, 41; social relationships and, 127; vocational, 142–44, 146, 158, *159–60*; wellness and, 22–25
Savci, M., 126
scapegoating, 2
scrapbooks, 200
second wave feminism, 3
secrecy, 103
secular organizations, 191
security, 106–7, 113
self, sense of, 12–13, 99, 151, 170, 184, 195
self-acceptance, 89–90, 137
self-care, 15, 99, 170
self-confidence, 77–79
self-consciousness, 167
self-control, 189–90
self-criticism, 63–64
self-discipline, 53
self-esteem, 107–8, 150
self-evaluation, 3
self-hatred, 14, 72
self-healing, 195
selfishness, 99, 165
self-judgments, 64
self-love, xiv, 99
self-motivation, 53, 167
self-reflection, 235
self-reinforcing, habits, 9
self-soothing behaviors, 18
self-sufficiency, 107
self-talk, negative, 64, 82
self-worth, 59, 82, 88, 151
sexism, 149
sexual abuse, 16–17, 107
sexual relationships, 17, 96, 98, 103
shame, 14, 17, 62–65, 72, 75, 92, 132, 183
shell metaphor, 105
shopping, clothing, 88
short term, 124; relationships, 111
sick days, 147–48
Simpa (friend), *145*, 154, 157–58
skiing, 163–64
skin, 77–78, 81, 84, 86–87, 89
sleep, 50, 65–67, 74
Sleep (journal), 65–66
SMART (specific, measurable, achievable, realistic, and timely) goals, 74–75, 178–79
smiling, 90
social capital, 152
social circle, 99, 118–20, *119*, 127, 139
social contract, 186, 190
social distancing, 8, 125
social media, 8–10, 51, *51*, 82, 117–18, *121*, 133–34, 136–37, 141, 166; addiction to, 11, 126. *See also specific social media*
social messages, 15–17
social networks, 118–20, *119*, 135–38
social relationships, socializing and, 18, 24–25, 167, 177; accessibility

and, 135–39; accountability and, 127, 130–33, 139; anonymity and, 133–35; exercises, 119, *119*, *121–22*; harmonious disagreement and, 128–30; loneliness and, 117–18; midlife, 122–24; societal changes impacting, 124–28; workplace, 144, 148, 156. *See also* intimate relationships
sociology, 15
sororities, for professional women, 123
the South, United States, 27–28, *51*, 163, 181
spirituality, spiritual health and, xvi, 24–25, 129, 181–83; "I Am" exercise and, 184, *184–85*. *See also* belief systems
stability, viii, 15, 48, 60–61
stages of realization, regarding aging and appearances, 83–91
stagnancy, xii–xiii
stamina, xiii, 58, 71–72, 84, 174
status quo, 87–88
Stellar, E., 59–60
stereotypes, 1
Stewart, Leslie, 169–71
stigmatization, 11, 188–89
stimulation, mental, 143
storge (love between parents and children), 98
Storyteller play personality, 169
stress, stressors and, 5, 21, 43–53, *50*, *51*, *52*, 111, 165; allostatic load and, 59–60; binge eating and, 8–9, 18; decision making and, 22; external, 40, 47–49, 60–61, 123–24; VUCA, 40, 43–45, 62; work related, 143, 146–47

strokes, 61
Structural Family therapy, 36–37
subjectivity, 36
suffering, 192
suffrage, for women, 187
sugars, 69–70
suicide hotline, United States, xvii
sun exposure, 67, 77, 86–87
sunscreen, 86–87
supermodels, 89
supernormal stimuli, 81–83
support networks, 137, 189–90
Sweeney, T. J., xv–xvi
swimming, 84
sympathetic nervous system, 22
sympathy, 55–56
systemic issues, 147

Taoism, 129
task-oriented activities, 165, 167
technology, 67, 77–79, 82, 118, 135–38
teenagers. *See* adolescence
telehealth, 39–40
temptation, 79
tension, feelings of, 12, 199
text messages, texting and, 117, 136
therapy, 36–37, 110, 154
Theresa (Mother), 188
thought blocking, 65
TikTok, 11
time, 8, 11, 35–36, 40, *101*; burnout and, 148; management, 154–55; personal, 174; physical health and, 58; social relationships and, 119, *119*, 124–25; in work-life balance, 141, 144–45, *145–46*, 149, *161*; worry, 65
to-do lists, 164, 166–67, 176

Torres, Dara, 84
toxic: relationships, 16, 106–12, 113–14, *114–15*, 116, *121*, 196; work cultures, 7, *121*, 143, 149–50
transactionality, 135–36
transmission, COVID-19, 44
trauma, wounds and, 16–17, 192–93, 196–97; belief system related, 184, 194–95
tropes, aging, 89–90
trust, 13, 49, 112, *121*, 192; forgiveness and, 186; transgressions of, 194–95
truth, xiv, 56, 93, 103–4

ubiquity of technology, 126, 137–38
ulterior motives, 127
uncertainty, 43–45, 48, 186
underrepresentation, 149
unemployment, 65
unequal pay, 149
unhappiness, 2, 5–7, 159
United States, xvii, 7, 97, 117–18, 147
universal ethics, 186–87
universities, 35, 83, 141–42
unpaid labor, 7
unplugging, from worklife, 156
unpredictability, 43, 59
Urban, Melissa, 155–56
urgency, *50*
US Department of Agriculture (USDA), 69

vagus nerve, 22
validation, 78–79, 93
value, self, xi, 200
values, 2, 18, 26–30, 41–42, 153, 167, 200–201; belief systems and, 14, 186, 193; conflicts in, 139; harmonious disagreement and, 128–30, 183; in intimate relationships, *101*, 101–2, *102*; physical health and, 57, 61, 72–75; in social relationships, *121–22*, 131–32; vocational satisfaction and, *159–60*; work-life balance and, 144–45, *145–46*, 149, *161*
vanity, 78
variant strains, COVID, 44
variety, 103–4
Verplanken, B., 64
video chats, real-time, 136
violations, boundary, 34
virtual worlds, online networks, 118, 125–27, 130–39; telehealth and, 39–40
vocations, 4–5, 24–25, 142–43, 151–59; burnout in, 142–44, 146–52, *160*; work-life balance in, 141, 144–45, *145–46*, 149, *161*, 162. *See also* workplace
volatility, 43–45, 48
volunteering, 191–92
voting, right of women to, 187
VUCA (volatility, uncertainty, complexity, and ambiguity) stressors, 40, 62
vulnerability, 65, 88, 96, 99, 104–5, 192; safety and, 105

weight, fluctuations in, 58, 63, 80–81
Welles, Orson, 26
wellness, well-being and, xv–xvi, 14, 21, 38; assessing, 22–25; belief systems and, 188–91; emotional, 41–42, 126; establishing a

baseline for, 25–26; eudaemonic, 165–67; leisure and, 165–67, 176; mental, xvii, 40–42. *See also* health

WFH. *See* working from home

white men, 188

white women, 3–4

WHO. *See* World Health Organization

widows, 97

willpower, 53

wisdom, 18, 73–75

women of color, 4

workaholic, 109

"work distress," 146

working from home (WFH), 125

work-life balance, 141, 144–45, *145–46*, 149, 154, *161*, 162

workplace: advancement opportunities, 149; boundaries, 33–36, 148, 154–56, 158; expectations, 155; leadership roles, 149, 152, 157; sabbaticals, 152; social relationships in the, 144, 148, 156

World Health Organization (WHO), 117–18, 146–47

worry time, 65

wrinkles, facial lines and, 77–78, 83–84, 87

Xennials, 4

Yoga Journal, 85–86

zoning out, 8, 166

ABOUT THE AUTHOR

Elizabeth O'Brien, PhD, LPC-MHSP, is a UC Foundation Professor at the University of Tennessee at Chattanooga and serves as the director of the School of Professional Studies in the College of Health, Education, and Professional Studies. Elizabeth has presented both internationally and nationally on issues related to wellness, marriage and couples counseling, and spiritual/ethical decision making. Dr. O'Brien maintains a small private practice in the Chattanooga area.